"Dr Anne Katz is THE expert for young adults struggling with the aftereffects of a cancer diagnosis. A must-have resource, this book belongs in the library of any parents or partners of young adult cancer patients and survivors."

Dan Dean, *founder of Cancer Dudes and non-Hodgkin's lymphoma survivor*

"The real-world conversations offered alongside professional recommendations set this book apart from others in its field and fill a very important gap in current literature. It is a must-read for anyone facing young adult cancer, either personally or professionally."

Mallory Casperson, *CEO + Founder, Cactus Cancer Society*

CARING FOR A YOUNG PERSON WITH CANCER

This book is an accessible, sensitive, and evidence-based resource for partners, parents, and other family members navigating the heartache and challenges of caring for a young adult with cancer.

When a young person you love is diagnosed with cancer, the impacts on partners and parents is life-altering. In this book, Anne Katz offers her unique perspective as a counselor to help family members as their child or partner goes through diagnosis, treatment, and the years of survivorship. Interweaving clinical practice with evidence-based tips and interventions, each chapter presents the story of a young person with cancer and how the illness impacts those that love them, with Dr. Katz providing gentle, targeted advice throughout. The chapters include individuals from diverse backgrounds, such as people across different ages, gender identities, ethnicities, and sexual orientations, as well as reflective questions, with topics covering treatment decision-making, how to care during treatment, letting go, and a resource section pointing readers to where they can seek help.

Written by a leading voice in the field of cancer, the stories and advice provided in this book will help all families and partners apply the lessons learnt to their lived experiences. It will be also of interest to health care providers working with these families, such as clinical social workers and nurses.

Anne Katz, PhD RN FAAN, is a certified sexuality counselor working with people of all ages who have cancer. She is the author of multiple books on cancer and sexuality.

CARING FOR A YOUNG PERSON WITH CANCER

Professional Guidance for Parents and Partners

Anne Katz

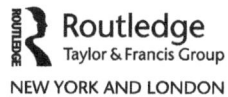

Routledge
Taylor & Francis Group

NEW YORK AND LONDON

Cover image: Getty

First published 2022
by Routledge
605 Third Avenue, New York, NY 10158

and by Routledge
4 Park Square, Milton Park, Abingdon, Oxon, OX14 4RN

Routledge is an imprint of the Taylor & Francis Group, an informa business

Library of Congress Cataloging-in-Publication Data
Names: Katz, Anne D., author.
Title: Caring for a young person with cancer: professional guidance for parents and partners / Anne Katz.
Description: New York: Routledge, 2022. | Includes bibliographical references and index. | Identifiers: LCCN 2021042993 (print) | LCCN 2021042994 (ebook) | ISBN 9781032151366 (hardback) | ISBN 9781032151359 (paperback) | ISBN 9781003242680 (ebook)
Subjects: LCSH: Cancer in adolescence. | Cancer in adolescence—Patients—Care. | Cancer—Patients—Family relationships. | Caregivers.
Classification: LCC RC281.C4 C394 2022 (print) | LCC RC281.C4 (ebook) | DDC 616.99/400835—dc23/eng/20211026
LC record available at https://lccn.loc.gov/2021042993
LC ebook record available at https://lccn.loc.gov/2021042994

ISBN: 9781032151366 (hbk)
ISBN: 9781032151359 (pbk)
ISBN: 9781003242680 (ebk)

DOI: 10.4324/9781003242680

Typeset in Joanna
by codeMantra

For my family

CONTENTS

1

INTRODUCTION

This book is for the people who love and support adolescents or young adults (AYAs) with cancer. AYAs have been called the 'lost tribe' because it is not always clear if they should receive treatment protocols for adults or children with cancer. But the parents and partners of these AYAs are perhaps the true lost tribe; there is nothing in their experience that has prepared them for this. While they stand behind next to their loved one, they are rarely the focus of support or help.

Cancer in Adolescents and Young Adults

Adolescence and young adulthood, between the ages of 15 and 39 years, is a stage of life unparalleled in physical, psychosocial, and cognitive growth. It is also a time when a significant number of developmental milestones need to be negotiated and attained in order to move into full adulthood. Physical growth includes changes in body composition, growth of organs, and production of sex hormones. Psychosocial growth includes the importance of the peer group rather than family, moving

DOI: 10.4324/9781003242680-1

from high school to college and eventual financial independence, and establishing romantic and sexual relationships. Cognitive growth allows for critical thinking, decision-making and planning for the future.

A diagnosis of cancer changes everything. Depending on the age and developmental stage of the person, achieving these milestones may be halted or delayed by the effects of treatment. Isolation from peers and reliance on parents impacts on gaining independence. This reliance may be practical, emotional, and/or financial. Career plans may be put on hold and uncertainty and fear of the unknown may replace plans for the future. Adolescents with cancer experience delays in graduation from high school and attendance at college. Those who are between the ages of 18 and 25 years may see interruptions in higher education and/or employment leading to lack of financial independence. They are also less likely to live independently of their parents than their peers and their social skills may fall below those of their peers. Those between 25 and 39 years of age may experience problems meeting potential partners, establishing long-term relationships, as well as sexual problems and fertility challenges. Depression and anxiety are common in this population and loss of self-esteem may occur as a result of all these psychosocial impacts.

These young people need specialized care when treated for cancer due not only to their physical health but especially for their emotional and psychosocial needs. Many of the side effects of treatment have unique consequences for young people; changes to the body from scars, weight gain or loss, and other physical changes may impact on their confidence that they are attractive and worthy of a romantic or sexual relationship. Isolation from the peer group may result in friends moving on with careers and relationships, leaving the young person with cancer feeling alone.

Delayed or late diagnosis of cancer is not infrequent in this age group. The person may not know that they should seek medical care, and when they do, health care providers may not suspect cancer as this is relatively rare in this age group. Symptoms of cancer such as fatigue or weight loss may be attributed to life style factors like late nights or poor diet. These delays may result in cancer being diagnosed at a late stage with poor outcomes. But cancer is one of the top 5 leading causes of death in AYAs.

Adolescents (15–19 years) are more commonly diagnosed with hematologic cancers as well as brain cancer. Young adults (aged 19+ years) experience breast, colorectal, thyroid, and melanoma more commonly. Treatment for cancer inevitably results in side effects that have impacts on quality of life. AYAs with cancer have overall poorer physical and mental health, and worse body image than their healthy counterparts.

Brain development continues until age 30 and the negative impact of cancer and its treatment on coping skills leads to a range of challenges including not following treatment regimens, missed appointments, and risky behavior (such as substance use). This is particularly important in adolescents who may have a lack of control/inhibitions and high needs for reward. This is not a conscious process but rather a function of brain development. Parental involvement may be necessary to ensure that the AYA attends for ongoing care and takes medication as prescribed, but this may be felt by the young person as controlling and intrusive, setting up the potential for conflict even though the parent(s) is doing what is best for their child. Evaluating the family structure, culture, and heritage as well as communication and interactions between the AYA with cancer and family members is an important part of holistic care and should be a part of the oncology team's focus.

Supporting the AYA with Cancer

So how can a parent or partner support the AYA with cancer? For some families, conflict and distancing may be present when a child is diagnosed with cancer. This may be an opportunity to mend the relationship but for some families, the rift may be too deep to reconnect. But in most families, the diagnosis draws people together and the support they give provides benefit to all.

When asked, AYAs with cancer want support but how that is provided is important. They want someone to be with them and stand by their side as they go through diagnosis and treatment. That person could be a partner, a family member, or a friend. This person can fulfil many different aspects of support such as attending appointments with the AYA and taking notes, and by providing emotional and financial support. Talking with and not telling the AYA what to do is seen as creating trust; the young person's involvement in any conversation must be voluntary and respectful with the supporter not claiming any power over the AYA by telling them what to do. Feeling that there is no judgment and that the parent is not talking down to them allows for sharing of feelings. Honesty is important and speaking in a direct manner is appreciated by AYAs with cancer. Parents may unconsciously be overprotective and their worry may result in treating the AYA as they would a much younger child. This is called 'infantalizing' and may manifest in different ways such as trying to control who the AYA socializes with or monitoring behavior. Parents have been known to forbid a young adult from dating or starting a sexual relationship; this is motivated by fear that something bad will happen to their YA child physically or emotionally.

AYAs are concerned about being a burden, so unconditional support and verbal assurances that being with them is not a burden is essential. They also want to be in control of information related to their cancer so asking before sharing news with other people is important for trust. They also want to be treated the same as they were before; being seen as strong or on the flipside, as being weak and in need of care, is not appreciated.

For both parents and partners, the diagnosis comes as a shock for which no one is ever prepared. A frequent thought – this should not be happening – encapsulates the changes in the present and future for both the AYA with cancer and their family members. A child of any age should not have to experience the challenges of a life-threatening illness and they should never die before their parent(s). Likewise, a young adult partner is never prepared to face the potential loss of their partner, or the challenges presented by treatment, hospitalization, and destruction of the plans they dreamed about.

Parents and partners may not have adequate support for their own needs. Larger academic cancer centers may have support groups and/or counselling for them but if the AYA is being treated in a smaller city or town, or in a private oncology practice, such support may not be available. The anxiety related to having a loved one with cancer can be overwhelming; finding help by talking to your primary care provider may be useful. Seeing a psychologist or other mental health care provider can be helpful if you are feeling depressed or anxious. You may need medication or ongoing counselling to help you while you do the hardest things you have ever had to do.

It is important for caregivers to attend to their own needs and seeking support from family members and friends may be a first step. "What can I do to help"? is a question often asked by others who genuinely want to help but may not know how or what help is needed. The parent/partner may not know what to respond so it's a good idea to think of some practical ways that others can do to lighten the load. Perhaps help can come in the form of doing laundry, watering the garden, or walking the dog; this time can be used by the caregiver to have a rest, do some physical exercise, or go to the hairdresser or any other task that needs to be done. Self-care has both physical and emotional components; physical exercise can help to alleviate mild to moderate depression and meditation helps to mitigate anxiety. Both of these activities cost little to nothing and pay dividends that can help you to support your child or partner.

Why Read This Book?

The chapters in this book describe common experiences of AYAs with cancer in their relationships with parents and partners and vice versa. There is nothing in life that prepares a parent or partner for cancer in their loved one. No matter how old or young you are and no matter how young or old your child or partner is, cancer changes everything.

You do not have to read every chapter in this book but you may learn something from each. Cancer is unpredictable and what you will go through as you support your child or partner is also unpredictable. You will find guidance from the description of what happened to the families in the chapters of the book. Each chapter tells the story of one family, one young person with cancer, and the parents and/or partner of that person.

All the people in these chapters are fictional. I hope the telling of the stories will be helpful to you as you face this challenge of caring for a loved one with cancer.

What You Will Find in the Pages of This Book

Each chapter in this book tells the story of one adolescent or young adult with the focus on the parent(s) and/or partner who are affected. Relationships are never perfect, and you will read about supportive parents and also those who get in the way of what the AYA needs as well as the partner who has all the best intentions but may not know what to do.

Chapter 2 describes the experience of a family with a 15-year old son who is diagnosed with sarcoma, a cancer of the soft tissues. The parents disagree on certain aspects of his care and the adolescent is stuck in the middle.

Chapter 3 describes the experience of a young adult diagnosed with malignant melanoma. The family struggles and asks for a second opinion, appearing to disregard the wishes of their daughter. The young woman with cancer decides that she wants to be part of the treatment decision-making process; this gives her some control, something that is important for any person with cancer.

Chapter 4 tells the story of a 17-year old with acute leukemia. In the process of having a stem cell transplant, his mother becomes over-protective and this impacts on her relationship with her son and his father. The mother is terrified that the treatment will not be successful, and her fear results in irrational behavior.

Chapter 5 describes the experience of a young couple who have to negotiate a new relationship with their parents after the woman has breast cancer. Relationships with family members and friends can be stressed by a cancer diagnosis and their need for care and support.

Chapter 6 highlights the experience of a 17-year old young man who ignores follow-up care after being treated for testicular cancer. He longs for life to be normal and in the process, terrifies his parents who are unaware that he has avoided follow-up care.

In Chapter 7 you will read about a same sex couple where one has an incurable brain cancer. Despite having legal documentation with instructions about who will make decisions for him when he is no longer able to, his parents intervene and want ongoing treatment against his wishes. Tensions emerge and accelerate between the man's parents and his husband as his condition worsens.

In Chapter 8 you will read about some of the struggles of parenting an adolescent. Adolescence is a time of rapid emotional and physical growth. Parents are often not prepared for the emotional changes that occur, not only for their child but also for the parent-child relationship. This normal event is even more challenging when a child has cancer.

Chapter 9 deals with one of the milestones of young adulthood. Finding a partner can be challenging after cancer. Parents can be seen to be interfering in this process with unwanted advice about dating and relationships. For young adults with a partner, the focus of returning to a 'normal' relationship includes their sexual relationship as well as having children in the future.

Chapter 10 highlights how family members often try to be the 'information finders' for the person with cancer, and this can lead to misinformation if they don't use reliable sources. There are many different organizations and associations that provide support for people with cancer and their families; these include providing valid information to financial assistance and also emotional and practical support. A list of resources is provided at the end of the chapter.

2

THE DIAGNOSIS

"OUR WORLD HAS TURNED UPSIDE DOWN"

Brad and Jillian Waters sat silently in the oncologist's office. Their son Josh sat next to his mother, his eyes focused on his clenched hands in his lap. His hands shook a little and Jillian reached across to touch them; he pulled away from her and gave her the kind of look only an adolescent can do with such effect. Jillian's eyes filled with tears and she quickly turned her face toward Brad.

Where was the doctor and why was it taking so long?

The door to the office opened and two people entered; the oncologist, Dr Steadman was tall with broad shoulders and messy hair and he apologized for the delay as he sat down behind the desk. A young woman followed close behind him. She smiled at the Waters family and then discovered that there was not a chair for her. She seemed a bit flustered and excused herself to go and find one. Before she returned, Dr Steadman cleared his throat and started to speak.

"I'm afraid it's not good news…"

Jillian took in a deep breath and Brad grabbed her hand.

DOI: 10.4324/9781003242680-2

"Josh", the oncologist looked at the 15-year old who was now looking at him with wide eyes and a deep flush on his cheeks, "As we suspected, you have sarcoma, a type of soft tissue cancer. This type of cancer happens in teenagers and young adults and while it is slow growing, we have to treat it as soon as possible to prevent it growing anymore."

"Hang on a minute there doc"!

Dr Steadman looked at the teenager's father who was now standing behind his chair. His wife grabbed his arm and forced him to sit back down.

"How can this have happened? My kid, he's an athlete! He plays football and tennis and is really fit! I wish I was as healthy! And there's no history of cancer in our family either! How can this happen"?

The oncologist listened as Brad spoke. By now the young woman had come back into the room, pushing an office chair on wheels against the wall where she sat down quietly.

"Mr and Mrs Waters, this is Angie Martin. She's a nurse navigator who works with families when a child is diagnosed with cancer. She will be with you every step of the way as Josh goes through treatment".

At the word 'treatment', Josh's head shot up. He'd been touching the area where the lump in his leg was, just above his right knee. The thought of having treatment had never entered his mind. Yes, he'd had an x-ray and then a CT scan, and finally an MRI. Someone had also stuck a needle into the lump to take out some fluid, but nobody had said anything more about it, until now. He thought that the pain in his leg was from an injury that happened last year when he was tackled on the football field.

What was the doctor talking about?

He looked at his parents; his mom's face was white, and she was crying. His dad was flushed, and he seemed angry.

"This is a lot to take in", the doctor continued, "The next step is for Josh to see an orthopedic surgeon who will remove the tumor. Based on what the pathologist says after examining the tissues, we will know if Josh needs further treatment. Do you have any questions"?

The Waters had a lot of questions but neither of them could find the words.

"I have a question", Josh's voice was a little wobbly and he was trying hard not to cry, "Am I going to ... are they going to... cut my leg off"?

Dr Steadman leaned over the desk to get closer to the young man.

"That is highly unlikely, Josh" his voice was soft but clear, "Your tumor, the lump, is not very big and we hope that it can be removed completely. The specialist I am sending you to will explain more. You are going to need to have surgery and we hope that this is all you will have to go through."

Jillian stood up suddenly.

"I'm sorry, but I have to get some air! Brad, Josh, let's go. I'm sorry Dr ….." She could not remember the doctor's name, "I can't process anything more right now. Can we come back and see you another time"?

Dr Katz advises:

Hearing the words 'you have cancer' is life changing for anyone, and when this is your child, not matter how young or old they are, this changes everything and your world will never be the same.

We know that after you hear those words, it is very difficult to hear anything else you are told; it's as if a train or strong wind is going through your brain. Research suggests that you hear only 10% of what you are told after hearing those words.

It is important that you have as many opportunities as you need to talk to the team who will be treating the cancer so that you have accurate information and get your questions answered in a way that makes sense to you.

In answer to her question, Angie the nurse navigator, spoke.

"I will be with you as you move through the treatment. Here is my business card; you can call or email me at any time. I will come to any appointments Josh has if you want and I am here to explain the medical language you will hear and answer any questions. If I don't know the answer, I will find someone who does. I will also be the one letting you know about upcoming tests and appointments".

The family walked through the door without acknowledging the doctor. It was Josh who led them to the lobby and exit of the cancer center. His parents seemed dazed and he found that almost amusing. They were always telling him what to do and how to act, and now he was the only one who seemed to keep it together.

The car ride home was silent. Josh listened to music on his phone and his father turned off the radio. Nobody said a word when they reached the house and Josh went straight to his room. He wanted to talk to someone, but who?

Jillian and Brad stood in the kitchen as if they didn't know what to do next. Brad tried to put his arms around his wife, but she moved away from him and ran up the stairs to their bedroom. Brad heard the door slam; was this how it was going to be? Both of them alone with their thoughts and Josh, the one who was most affected, separate and out of reach?

> Dr Katz advises:
> Everyone processes information differently and your initial response to the diagnosis does not predict how you will feel and act in the future. Josh, as many adolescents do, wants to talk to a friend, perhaps to tell them what has happened or just to act as if nothing is wrong. Jillian has reacted to this news emotionally, and she needs to be by herself, perhaps to protect her husband from her overwhelming feelings. Brad had tried to hug his wife but was rebuffed; this might be a reflection of who he is, someone needing the comfort of a hug as much as he thinks his wife does. Every family and every individual family member will react differently; there is no right or wrong way to do this.

The next day Angie called to check in with the family. Brad didn't want to talk, and Jillian kept the call brief. Yes, they were doing okay and no, they weren't ready to discuss this further, they just needed time to adjust. Angie agreed to only contact them with information about the next appointments and they would contact her if they needed anything.

She sent them an email the next day that Josh had an appointment with the orthopedic surgeon at the end of the week. Angie offered to go with them, but Jillian responded that they would be fine going without her. When she told Brad about the appointment he asked if Angie would be there. He was annoyed that Jillian had responded to the nurse navigator without talking to him first. When she told Josh about the appointment, he was quiet for a moment and then he too asked if Angie was going to be there. Now Jillian felt guilty about what she had done. She had been looking for information on the internet and thought she knew what needed to be done about Josh's treatment so why did they need another person in the room? What she had read seemed pretty clear cut. Josh would have the surgery and that was the end of it. What else could Angie add to the information the oncologist had given them?

On Friday at 1 pm they found themselves waiting to see the orthopedic surgeon. Thirty minutes later they still had not been called and Brad was getting annoyed. Josh had his ear buds in and was listening to something at full volume; his mother could hear the 'whomp whomp' of the techno music he liked, and this was irritating. Why did he need the volume to be so loud? She had warned him about the long-term effects on his hearing, but of course he didn't listen to her.

Almost 45 minutes later they were shown to an examination room and they waited there for another ten minutes until a young woman entered the room. She introduced herself as the intern working with Dr Bennett the surgeon. She asked what seemed to be hundreds of questions and Josh answered them. Jillian wanted to add more details, but the intern seemed satisfied with Josh's 'yes', 'no' and 'kinda' responses. She thanked them and left the room without telling them when Dr Bennett might arrive.

Another doctor came into the room ten minutes later. He introduced himself as Dr Bennett's 'fellow' and he also asked a lot of questions, some of them a repeat of what the intern had asked. Brad grew more and more irritated, and Jillian shot him a look that clearly told him to keep quiet. This doctor examined Josh's knee; he poked and prodded and Jillian could see that this was painful for Josh. She wanted to tell him to stop, but she knew this was necessary. Finally, the surgeon entered the room. He was a large man wearing scrubs and a cotton cap on his head. He looked rushed and apologized as he sat down on a stool near the examination table.

"Sorry for the delay ... I got called to the OR for an emergency. Horrible car crash on the highway..."

Dr Katz advises:

Academic hospitals usually have trainees of various levels who see the patient before the specialist does. They take the history of the illness and do an initial physical examination. This can seem a waste of time and also a repetition of questions, but they need to learn, and they pass on the information from the patient and the examination to the specialist.

Delays are quite common as emergencies happen and require the specialist to deal with urgent cases; this is annoying when you are waiting anxiously to be seen.

It's a pity that the nurse navigator was not with them as she could have provided an explanation for the delay and could have talked to the family about what to expect from the visit with the surgeon and distracted them while they waited. Not all cancer centers or hospitals have nurse navigators; that's a pity because they really help patients and families.

The surgeon examined the area above Josh's knee where the lump was. His hands were large, but he was gentle. He then showed the images from the CT scan and MRI and explained to the family what he thought he would do in the surgery. Josh looked at the scans intently; it was cool to see his bones, white against the black background, and the tumor was clearly visible. The surgeon's voice came in and then went out of his hearing. He heard the words 'early stage' and 'we'll have to see what the pathology shows'; his mother kept interrupting the doctor and Josh tried to tune her out. Then there was quiet, and Josh looked away from the images on the computer. Was someone asking him something?

"Hey buddy", his father's voice was too loud, "Did you hear what the doctor asked you"?

Josh looked at the doctor who had a small smile on his face.

"Those images are pretty interesting, right? I asked if you understood what was going to happen", the doctor's voice was soft, and it seemed weird to Josh that such a big man would have such a gentle voice.

"Uh, maybe I didn't hear exactly what you said. Sorry..."

"No problem. Here it is again. The tumor in your leg is about 2 cm by 1 cm, that's less than one inch long and about a half an inch wide. I think it will be a fairly simple surgery to take it out, but you might need some tissue grafting to fill in the hole where the growth was. We won't know more until the pathologist looks at the tumor under the microscope and can give us a report about the grade of the cancer. Does that make sense to you"?

There were some words that Josh didn't really understand, but he didn't want to seem stupid, so he just nodded his head.

The surgeon apologized again as he left the room.

"I have to go back to the OR ... more victims of that car crash to see to. My assistant will send you information about when you'll have the surgery and details about tests before..."

And with that, he was gone. The three of them sat for a while. What were they supposed to do? Was someone else coming to see them? What about the other doctors they had seen before the surgeon, the ones who asked all the questions? After ten tense minutes where Brad got more and more irritated, they left.

Almost as soon as they drove into the garage, Jillian's cell phone rang; it was Angie the nurse navigator. She was calling to hear how the appointment with the surgeon went. Jillian hesitated before pressing the speaker button so that the rest could hear.

Before she could say anything, Josh spoke up.

"I kinda wish you'd been there. I'm not sure I heard everything right and well, I guess I need to know what's going on so that I can understand what's going to happen".

Jillian looked shocked. The surgeon had been very clear in her opinion, and she thought that they all understood what was going to happen.

"I agree with Josh," Brad said in a firm voice, "I want to be sure I heard everything too. My mind was going a mile a minute and I might have missed something. Can we meet with you again"?

"Of course we can meet again! This is why I'm here, to help you navigate the system and that includes making sure that you have all the information that you need. How does Monday morning sound? We can meet before Josh needs to be at school and you need to be at work. How does 7:30 sound"?

Josh stifled a groan; he hated getting up early and his Dad was not much better. His mom was an early bird so the time should not be a problem for her.

"Um, that seems a bit early for me…" Jillian said, her voice sounded angry to both Brad and Josh.

"It's fine," Brad said, giving his wife a stern look, "We'll be there on time. Can you give us directions from the lobby of the cancer center to where your office is"?

Josh went into this room and started playing a video game. The sound of tires screeching and horns blaring coming from the computer drowned out the raised voices of his parents in the study downstairs.

"Why are you acting this way? I don't understand why you are so opposed to this Angie person! She's here to help us!" Brad's voice grew louder until he was almost shouting.

"Can you keep your voice down? Josh can hear you! I don't want to upset him anymore that he already is!"

Jillian's voice was also loud, but she didn't seem to notice.

"I don't know why we have to involve another person in this! Both doctors have been very clear; he needs to have the surgery and that's that. Why do you have to question every damn thing I say?"

"YOU may have this straight in your head, but I don't! I think Angie could be a great help for ALL of us. But you are so darn stubborn! It's always your way or the highway and this time it's not going to work! This is our kid, not just yours!"

Brad's heart was pounding; he had never been so angry with her in the almost 21 years they had been married.

"Do you think I don't know that he's YOUR kid too? I just have to look at his face to see your image! I just want to keep this between us! I don't want strangers in our business! I understood the doctors perfectly! I can't help it if you are too dumb to understand this too…"

As she shouted the last sentence, she realized she had said something that she couldn't take back. Her face was flushed, and she tried to touch his shoulder, but he pushed her away and stormed out the house. She heard the car door slam and the engine start and then the sound of metal, BOOM!, as he reversed into the closed garage door.

Josh ran down the stairs, his headphones around his neck and the cord swinging across his chest.

"What have you done, Mom??? Is Dad okay?"

Dr Katz advises:

Because individuals have different ways of dealing with difficult situations, there may be conflict about anything related to the plans for treatment or other matters. It is not uncommon for couples to try to cope the best way they know how, and to not understand why the other person is not doing what they are, or just doing things differently.

The way we communicate during stressful times or in an argument can make the situation worse. Both Brad and Jillian are using 'you' in their communication and this results in a defensive response from the other who feels accused. Using 'I' statements puts the emphasis on what YOU are feeling rather than putting those feelings on the other person. Losing one's temper as Jillian did led her to calling her husband 'stupid', something that is both insulting and likely not true at all. Words said in anger will lead to hurt feelings and sometimes irreversible damage to the relationship.

Brad was fine, his ego was a bit hurt, but he and Jillian knew that this accident was as a result of his anger and distress. The car bumper could be fixed, and the garage door would likely have to be replaced. It was a wake-up call for them both; they needed to be united as they faced the future for Josh that was scary and uncertain. After reassuring Josh that he was fine, Brad suggested that he and his wife go for a walk and talk about what was happening.

As they walked through the neighborhood, they talked openly about how they were feeling. Jillian admitted that she was in Mamma Bear mode, and that seeking out information on the internet helped her to feel in control. Brad told her that he was terrified and didn't know what to do to protect Josh; this was a new experience for him and one that he had no idea how he could deal with. Soon they were holding hands as they walked, and Jillian even managed to smile at a little girl who was watering the lawn and most of the driveway of a house around the corner from their home. They talked about her reluctance to have Angie, the nurse navigator, involved in Josh's care. Brad expressed how he felt about having someone to help them now and in the future, and that he hoped it would take some of the pressure off them to find information. Jillian was still hesitant, but she agreed to try for a couple of weeks, and if she felt it wasn't working for her to have Angie involved, they would figure out something together. They returned home feeling lighter and more connected.

That night they asked Josh to sit with them for a while after dinner. He usually left the table after inhaling whatever was on his plate, but he wanted to talk to them too.

"Josh, we're sorry you heard us arguing", Brad began. "It's just that, well, we're in shock I guess, and we hadn't really talked about this ourselves and obviously not with you".

"And after the garage door incident, we went for a walk and we talked about how we are feeling. And then we realized that we don't know how YOU are feeling. We're so sorry, Josh, we really haven't done anything right in this whole thing".

Jillian was crying openly now, and Brad took her hand.

"I guess I don't really know how I'm feeling," answered Josh, "I hate to see you guys fighting and it's all my fault…"

"Hang on here, buddy", Brad interrupted his son, "This is NOT your fault. None of this is your fault. This is a horrible thing that has happened to YOU and we should be the adults in this. Instead we have been acting stupidly and haven't given you the support you need".

"And that changes right now!" Jillian had stopped crying and was back in Mamma Bear mode. "We promise you that we will not fight about this again and we promise that we will support you in whatever way we can…"

"Maybe it's the way Josh wants", Brad suggested, "He's 15 years old and this is his body. Maybe we should be following his lead…"

Jillian smiled briefly. "But he's still my baby, my only baby".

"Jeesh, Mom, I'm not a baby! I've told you that a million times! And I do want your support – I know I am going to need it. But the way I see it, I don't really have a choice right now. The lump or tumor or whatever has to come out. I have to get through this, and I will. You also".

His parents looked at each other and then at him: when did he get to be so mature?

"And another thing. I like that Angie person. She's there to help us so why cut her out? Let's go on Monday even though it's the most awful time. If we don't think that she can help us, then we don't need to see her again. Okay? For my sake?"

Dr Katz advises:

An adolescent may be old enough to participate in their care plan and certainly should have a voice in any decisions that have to be made. A parent's desire to protect their child is natural, but ultimately, the treatment happens to the adolescent. Adolescents progress through this stage of life in their own time and at their own speed. Some are still immature at the age of 15, but Josh is showing a great deal of maturity in dealing with his upcoming surgery.

The developmental tasks of adolescence include achieving independence, separating from parents, and gaining autonomy. Cancer tends to mature adolescents and so it is important to encourage them to be involved in treatment planning. It is also important to recognize that as a parent, no matter how distressed you are, this is happening to your child and they have the right to agree to what is being done to them. To try to protect them, although a natural impulse, is in the end not helpful and may even be detrimental to their emotional health.

On Monday morning, the three of them met with Angie. For the first ten minutes she explained what her role was and how she could support them in any way that they wanted. She provided them with written information as well as explaining the various support groups that they could join as parents with a child with cancer, and some online support groups for Josh that focused on adolescents with cancer. She explained that because sarcoma is fairly rare, there were not specific in-person support groups for people diagnosed with sarcoma, but he would find other people with the same kind of cancer in the national support groups.

Jillian was still quite reserved during the meeting; she didn't say much but at least she didn't roll her eyes as Brad feared she would. About halfway through their time together, Angie asked Josh if he would like to speak to her alone, without his parents in the room.

"Oh, that won't be necessary…" Jillian started to say but Josh cut her off.

"That would be great, Thanks".

"Of course, that's fine, buddy" said Brad as he tugged at his wife's arm, "We'll meet you outside. Take your time…"

Josh looked a little embarrassed as they left.

"Excuse my mom, she's been a little … um, stressed by this".

"I bet she has," replied Angie, "So, how can I help you? I bet you have a million questions".

And he did.

The day of the surgery arrived. They were all up earlier than they needed to be, and Josh thought his mom must not have slept at all. In fact, she looked really awful. But then he did too; he had glanced at himself in the mirror after his shower and his eyes were bloodshot. He had spent most of the night listening to music, switching from the techno he preferred to something more soothing that he hoped would help him fall asleep. It hadn't worked that well but here he was, ready to do what had to be done. His Dad looked fine unless he focused on his shoulders that appeared about three inches higher than they normally were. He was stressed, Josh could see that right away but he chose to not comment about that, or about his Mom.

Angie was waiting for them in the lobby of the hospital. She walked with them to the admissions office, waited while Josh checked in, and then showed them the way to the OR suite. She sat with them while they waited for Josh to be called; Jillian tried to hide her tears as they wheeled him through the double doors, the top of his head the last thing she saw as the doors closed. When she could no longer see her son, she cried openly. Brad was emotional too, he had tears in his eyes that he wiped away with the back of his hands. Angie put her arm around Jillian's shoulders, saying nothing as Josh's mother sniffed and wiped her nose on her sleeve.

In a scratchy voice Jillian whispered to the nurse navigator: "Thank you for being here, Angie. I, we, needed you."

Conclusion

In the aftermath of a diagnosis of cancer in their child, the parents may react with disbelief and in different ways, based on their separate personalities and coping mechanisms. It is not uncommon for one parent, often but not always the mother, to become hypervigilant and protective. This can cause conflict with the other parent and puts the young person right in the middle. Open and honest communication is vital to avoid this; each parent needs to allow the other to cope as well as they can but they also be supportive because there is no right or wrong way to deal with a child's illness, no matter how old or young they are.

Reflective Questions

- How could have Josh's parents handled the situation differently when the doctors asked so many questions?
- What should parents do when it seems as if their adolescent has not heard the same information that they did?
- How can parents avoid causing their child stress when they are in conflict?

3

TREATMENT
DECISION-MAKING

"HOW CAN WE HELP"?

Maddison ('Madds' to her friends and family) Walter is an outgoing 22-year old who finished college in the Spring and is excited about her new job as a copywriter at an independent publishing company that starts in a month. She was looking for an apartment in downtown Boston to be close to work while she was home now for a couple of weeks, back in her childhood bedroom with the double bed and one wall covered in photos from the many years she had spent at Camp Wapaloosa. Her parents, Ted and Carol, are thrilled to have her home, even for just a while. They had missed her terribly when she was away at college; they both would have preferred her to live at home now rather than in the apartment she had rented.

"I guess the commute from here to the job really is too long", sighed her mother as Maddison searched on her computer for an apartment close to the company where she was to work.

"Mom….. we've been through this a million times! I love you guys but I'm 22 and I've lived away for 4 whole years… and you keep on about

DOI: 10.4324/9781003242680-3

this! I'm going to do this, and it would make my time here much happier if you just stopped!"

Carol turned away from her daughter, hoping she didn't see the tears in her eyes. Why had she and Ted decided to have only one child? She didn't think about this often, but when she and Madds had 'words', the regrets entered her head. If only they had another child at home, she would not dread Maddison leaving…

Maddison suddenly stood up, her chair slamming into the kitchen cupboards.

"I'm late! Darn it! I have a hair appointment and I'm late!"

Before Carol could say goodbye, Maddison slammed the door shut behind her and then the car door slammed, and she was off.

She returned two hours later, and instead of showing off her new haircut, she was subdued. Ted and Carol looked at each other and Ted shrugged. After all the years of living with these two women, he still couldn't anticipate their response to pretty much everything. Maddison's hair looked great to him; the summer sun had not yet bleached her ginger curls and her hair shone in the late afternoon light. He loved that she had inherited his red hair, seemingly the only thing she had in common with him. She was so much like her mother in all other ways; her outgoing personality, almost constant cheerfulness, and love of all things natural.

"Is there some wine open? Or a beer?"

Maddison stood in front of the fridge, her back to her parents but they could see that something was wrong. She found a bottle of beer at the back of the lower shelf, twisted the cap off, and sat down. Without raising her eyes from the table, she told her parents what had happened. The hairdresser, someone she had never seen before, had noticed something on her scalp. She was shocked when he said that she needed to get it looked at. Maddison had asked how he knew this, and he told her that they were taught this during their training. He knew what to look for, but he also said that he was not a doctor and she should see someone as soon as possible.

Her parents were shaken. Ted went to see a dermatologist every year; when he was in his thirties, he had a couple of moles on his back removed, and Carol insisted that he get a full body skin check routinely. But they had neglected to do the same for Maddison, who with her red hair, fair skin, and freckles was also at risk. Within a few days Maddison had seen Ted's dermatologist and a biopsy was performed on the 'thing' on her scalp. The results came back within a week and it was bad. She had melanoma and she needed to have the 'thing', now called the 'lesion', removed in its entirety. She needed to see a plastic surgeon who would cut out the 'thing' on her head; she hoped she would not have a giant scar on her head after that. And after all that, she needed to see an oncologist who would recommend treatment.

She went to the plastic surgeon who removed the lesion; it hurt a lot afterward. There was a two-week wait before she could see the oncologist and Maddison spent most of the time in her bedroom with the door closed. Her parents were devastated and wanted to speak to her, but the door remained shut. They heard her late at night as they were getting ready for bed; the fridge door opened and closed, cutlery rattled, and then the back door closed softly. They thought they smelled smoke when she was out there but that couldn't be possible! Madds was so health conscious and she would never smoke anything.

The day of the appointment arrived, and Maddison was surprised when she found her parents dressed and waiting to accompany her to see the oncologist.

"What are you doing?" she blurted out. "You're not coming with me to this appointment. I'm going alone".

"Oh no, you are definitely NOT going alone, young lady!"

Her father's voice was shaky. He hardly ever spoke loudly but this time was different.

"We are coming with you and that's that. I mean it, Maddison…"

He never called her Maddison and she relented. Maybe them coming with her was not a bad idea; she didn't really know what to expect and in reality, she was really scared.

Dr Katz advises:

If possible, it is important for trusted others to accompany the person with cancer to all appointments. Four (or more) ears are always better than two and we know that it is difficult to take in all that is talked about at these appointments. The 'patient' may become over-loaded with the information presented and it can be almost impossible to listen and think about questions that need to be asked. The person (or people) who go with the young adult can take notes so that information is recorded for review later.

Many cancer centers also allow for audio recording of these appointments; all you have to do is ask if that is possible. And if family members cannot be present, ask if they can call in on their phone to listen to what is said and to have the opportunity to ask their own questions.

They drove in silence to the oncologist's offices in a nearby suburb. Carol, who had been looking at websites while they waited for this appointment, had been surprised that they were not going to a 'proper' cancer center in Boston. But this is where the dermatologist referred them so she would see how the appointment went.

Dr Paisley seemed too young to be an oncologist; Maddison's parents seemed a little shocked, but she felt confident that the doctor was not 'an old guy' as she later told her parents. It felt to Maddison that the doctor really knew her stuff and she took the time to explain exactly what needed to happen. The pathology report from the wide excision that the plastic surgeon had done was not back yet and the oncologist wanted to get a head start on other investigations; Maddison was going to need blood tests, and something called a sentinel node biopsy, and maybe a CT scan as well as an MRI. This would happen over the next few days at another facility and then she would have another appointment with Dr Paisley, and they would discuss treatment options. Maddison and her parents were introduced to Dallas, the physician assistant who worked with the oncologist. He explained his role and gave them each one of his business cards.

Maddison had all the tests and the sentinel node biopsy that hurt a LOT. She was annoyed that she had each on a different day; she was exhausted from driving back and forth to the imaging center. Both her parents had offered to go with her, but she needed the time to think about what was happening. Flashes of memory came and went as she drove to the imaging center. There was that summer at camp when she lost her hat and got a really bad sunburn. And the other time at college when she went away to a friend's place at the beach and forgot to use sunscreen and there was nowhere to buy any. But why was this thing on her head?

Dr Katz advises:

Melanoma is the most serious type of skin cancer and is associated with exposure to the sun or tanning beds. It can occur on the skin of the scalp where it often goes unnoticed by the person. Having fair skin, common in those with red hair, or having a bad sunburn are risk factors for developing a melanoma.

Investigations include a biopsy and/or removal of the lesion that is then looked at by a pathologist to assess how thick the melanoma is and if more tissue needs to be removed. A sentinel node biopsy is done to see if any cancer has spread to the lymph nodes and additional tests such as a CT or MRI scan may be ordered to see if there is spread to other areas of the body. Treatments for melanoma are based on these scans and pathological findings.

The next week, Maddison and her parents returned to the oncologist. Maddison was terrified that she would need chemotherapy or some other treatment. She knew that her mother had been researching this kind of cancer online and she had a notebook with her that no doubt contained a list of questions about a mile long. Maddison was actually happy about that; she'd been so busy having all those tests and her head still hurt where they cut out the lesion on her scalp and one lower down where they did the sentinel nose biopsy. She hadn't looked at the wound in the mirror and she kept her hair in a ponytail so that no one would see the wound on her scalp. The sentinel node biopsy spot was at the back of her neck close to her hairline and her ponytail hid that.

At the oncologist's office she sat with her parents in the waiting room for what seemed like hours but was just ten minutes before they were called to the oncologist's office. Dallas, the physician assistant, entered the room minutes later with a solemn look on his face. Maddison took a deep breath and glanced over at her parents; her mother looked like a ghost and her father was staring at a painting on the wall. The news was obviously not good.

Dr Paisley sat down at her desk and confirmed that the news was indeed not good. She started to talk about what would happen next, but Maddison did not hear anything. The oncologist went on and on and soon her words were just a background noise. When she eventually stopped talking, Carol put out her hand as if to stop the flow of words from the doctor.

"Dr Paisley", her mother's voice was a little too loud, "I... we, would like a second opinion from someone at an academic center. I don't mean to insult you but what you are proposing sounds really harsh and we need a second opinion..."

Maddison felt like she was on the edge of cliff; what was going to happen next? Why was her mother interfering? She was not sure what the oncologist had said but why did she need a second opinion? Was this going to make the oncologist angry with them and how would this impact on her treatment in the future? As she sat there, she realized that her parents were out of their seats and waiting for her at the door. She didn't know what to say to Dr Paisley, so she got up and followed her parents to the car. She was mortified.

Dr Katz advises:

Getting a second opinion can be helpful for many reasons and if a doctor refuses to send you to see someone else, this is a warning sign that you really do need to get another opinion about the diagnosis and/or treatment. A second opinion, if the recommendations are the same as the original physician, provide reassurance that the treatment that was recommended is the right one. Trust in the treating oncologist is known to lessen regrets about treatment plans, yet another reason to get a second opinion.

Maddison and her parents talked about what Dr Paisley had suggested; it all sounded horrible to her with more surgery and all sorts of chemotherapy. According to her mother, there were newer and more effective treatments available at the cancer center as well as all sorts of other supportive services.

"We want the very best treatment for you, Madds," she said, with tears in her eyes. Her dad nodded in agreement.

"But... what about the money? Am I covered by your insurance, Dad?" Maddison could hardly get the words out. She was not sure how much this would all cost, but she thought it would be a lot. At college she had been covered by student insurance, but did her parents even have health insurance and would she be included? Her head hurt thinking about this.

"Maddison", her father's voice was firm, "We will not talk about money now or ever. That is not an issue. Do you hear me? Not another word!"

He sounded angry, something rare for him, and Maddison excused herself and said she was going for a walk. Carol and Ted looked at each other as the door closed.

"I hope she's not going to smoke..." Carol's voice was a mix of frustration and concern.

"Just let it go, honey. We have a bigger fight to face... at this point, what is a cigarette or two?"

"I'll tell you, Ted, smoking is an absolute no go, especially now... I read that ..."

Ted just shook his head and pushed his chair back. He needed a break from all of this. From the worry and the fear and Carol talking to him like he was an idiot.

Dr Katz advises:
Every parent's worst nightmare is that their child, no matter how young or old, will get sick. How they deal with this can vary; some parents are united in their approach and support each other while also supporting their child. Other parents have different views on what should happen, and this may cause conflict and even separation/divorce. The impact of a cancer diagnosis in a child can bring some couples closer together or may drive some apart.

Two weeks later they drove to Boston to the cancer center. Maddison had cycled past it when she was at college, but it looked different now that she actually had to go inside. Her mother had asked for all the images and results from Dr Paisley's office and she carried them in a bright red folder. Maddison had not looked at them. She was still unsure why Dr Paisley was not good enough for her mother, but she was tired of fighting and she knew that her parents were arguing. She heard them late at night, through their bedroom door. Her mother sounded so angry and her dad seemed so withdrawn.

They spent the rest of the day there. They saw different physicians who each took the red folder, left the room for a while and then came back, often followed by a group of people Maddison's age and even younger. There were medical students, interns and residents as well as something called 'Fellows' although a few of them were young women. Their roles were explained to them by a woman who appeared to be a similar age to Carol and Ted. She had introduced herself to them as Angela and explained that she was the Clinical Nurse Specialist who worked with the doctors but was there to ensure that Maddison was supported.

"What about us?" thought Carol, "We need support too", but she didn't say this out loud. Carol felt much happier with the physicians at the cancer center. They seemed more on top of things and they seemed to be living up to their reputation as the best in the northeast.

The final appointment of the day was scheduled with the 'attending', Dr Phillips. Angela the 'special' nurse was there along with one of the Fellows who had not introduced himself to them. Dr Phillips looked imposing with his shiny bald head and well-groomed salt-and-pepper beard. But his eyes were kind and his voice soft as he started to speak. He looked directly at Maddison who wanted him to talk to her parents; she was afraid that like with Dr Paisley, she would tune him out. But Dr Phillips spoke in short chunks, stopping often to ask if she had any questions. Maddison could sense that her mother was getting a little impatient; she made a hissing sound as if she wanted to interrupt but Dr Phillips ignored her. "Poor Mom", Maddison thought, "she must be so frustrated!"

Dr Phillips stopped after about ten minutes; he had gone over the results of all the tests she had. There was cancer in one of the lymph nodes and while this was concerning, recent advances using something called targeted therapy had shown excellent results.

"Now Maddison, I have an important question for you".

Carol took this as an invitation to talk. "Excuse me, Dr Phillips but I want to ask something..."

"You must have lots of questions Mrs Walter, and there will be time for that when I have an answer to my question for your daughter".

His voice was firm, and Carol sat back in the chair.

"Maddison", he started with a serious look on his face, "What role do you want to play in your treatment plan? By that I mean how involved do you want to be in deciding what treatment to have. You have choices in this; you can leave those decisions to me and my team or you can play an active role in deciding what you want or don't want."

Maddison was shocked. The other oncologist had told her and her parents what the treatment would be and here was this doctor telling her she had a choice!

Dr Katz advises:

Young adults, and even some adolescents, have the capacity to understand the recommended treatment and should be involved in making a decision about the plan. These decisions are on a spectrum from deciding alone what treatment they agree to or can be shared with the cancer care team or leaving treatment decisions completely in the hands of the cancer care team. Trust in the treating oncologist is known to lessen regrets about treatment plans, yet another reason to get a second opinion.

A study has shown that most young adults want a shared approach with some wanting limited involvement of parents. Treatment regret is not uncommon, and this can have a long-lasting effect on dealing with side effects of treatment and quality of life.

Maddison thought about this for a couple of minutes. She was exhausted, partly because she had started to wake up in the middle of the night and could not get back to sleep. The wound on her scalp was still painful and she could not get comfortable. In the dark her mind would go to places that terrified her. What if the cancer couldn't be cured? What did he mean by 'targeted therapy'? Her thoughts bounced around, and she could sense her mother's eyes on her.

"Umm… I guess… maybe you should just tell me what to do?"

This was all she could say in the moment; she looked across at her father who was staring at her with a confused look on his face.

"Dad?" her voice shook, "Is that not what I should do? I don't know what to do"!

Her father's voice was strong and clear in response to her.

"Madds, this is your decision to make, along with the professionals of course. You are strong and smart, and this is YOUR life. It's not easy, I understand, but you're an adult and you have to go through the treatments. We are here to support you, but we cannot experience whatever you are going to go through with the treatments".

His assurances and calm advice helped Maddison to gain some control in the moment.

"Okay, my Dad's right. I want to know more – about the treatments and the side effects – and then I'll decide".

Dr Phillips smiled and held out his hand to her.

"We're partners in this, Maddison. Nothing will happen without a full explanation and time for you to decide. Angela, the CNS, uh… clinical nurse specialist, is going to be your closest ally for the next months. Now, let me explain what I propose, and you tell me what you think…"

Carol interrupted again.

"Can we have some time to talk about this, please? This has been a lot to take in and well, we came her for a second opinion…"

The look on Maddison's face stopped Carol.

"Sure, Mrs Walter, take all the time you want. We'll leave now and will come back once you've had a break". Dr Phillips motioned for the Fellow to leave the office.

"Maybe you'll be more comfortable at the coffee shop in the lobby", suggested Angela. "I need something to drink and I'll be in shouting distance in case you have a question and then I can show you the way back when you're done. Make sense?"

Maddison smiled at the nurse; she was 100% right. She needed to talk to her parents and her mom needed to listen to her. She knew her Dad would go along with what she decided, but her Mom needed to calm down. This place felt right. Dr Phillips seemed really smart and Angela had already shown that she understood the family. The thought of being able to make decisions gave her a sense of control and that felt good.

They followed Angela into the elevator in silence. There were posters on the walls of the elevator showing a variety of classes that patients could sign up for. There were all kinds of yoga, support groups, and a wellness center where massages and guided meditation sessions took place. Maddison stared at them and she tugged on Ted's sleeve to prompt him to read what was available. He had noticed them too and squeezed her hand.

They found an empty table and Ted asked them what they wanted to drink and went to get them coffee. Angela sat down at another table; she was close enough to the family that they could call her over if they needed to.

Maddison took a deep breath.

"Why did you say that we were only here for a second opinion, Mom? This was YOUR idea in the first place! I was SO embarrassed! It was like you didn't trust them!"

Her voice had risen, and she sounded like she was about to cry. Ted had returned and he put his hand over hers on the table.

"Honey, it's okay. Let's just talk this through. Give your Mom a chance to explain…"

Maddison looked at her mother who was paging through her notebook as if looking for some sort of universal truth.

"Mom?"

Carol opened her mouth to speak but instead started to sob. Maddison looked confused for a moment and then reached over to hug her. They sat like this for a while and Carol stopped crying and blew her nose.

"Thanks, Madds. I'm sorry… this is not what you need right now but it's just hit me. This is real, it's not a bad dream… my poor baby…. I just want to make this all go away…"

Dr Katz advises:

It is natural to want to take away the hurt and pain of your child. And all parents would rather experience this than have their child go through what lies ahead. Some degree of denial (it just hit me, this is not a bad dream) is usual and a way of coping. But in the end, parents cannot take away the reality of a cancer diagnosis and what that means. While it is a terrible thing to face, a parent has to face what has happened and be there to support the young adult, putting themselves second to the needs of their child.

Maddison couldn't help smiling; her Dad had a grin on his face too that he quickly hid as his wife looked at him. When would she act like Madds was, in fact, 22 and had been living away from them for four whole years and had done fine?

"Madds", Carol began with a little wobble in her voice, "The reason that I thought this was just a second opinion and not the final decision about treatment is because, I guess, I just didn't want this to be real. Do you know what I mean?"

Maddison nodded. She didn't want it to be real either, but it was and the sooner she started treatment, the sooner it would be over.

"Mom, this was YOUR idea in the first place and I'm so grateful! You did all that reading while I shut myself in my room. And it was YOU who suggested that we come here. And just think about how today has gone..."

This time Carol nodded, and Maddison saw that her father had tears in his eyes.

"This place is AMAZING, Mom. Dr Phillips talked about all the research they're doing, and the other doctor didn't mention that AT ALL! And she didn't talk about these new drugs! She only talked about MORE surgery and chemotherapy! And then there's Angela! And that other guy, the cute one... what's his name again?"

"Maddison!" her mother sounded shocked, "I think his name is Dallas and he's here to help you along with the rest of them! And do you really think he's cute?"

"C'mon you two!" Ted had a smile on his face, but his voice was serious. "We're supposed to be talking about other stuff! Maddison, are you happy to start treatment here?"

"Yes! Yes!" Maddison sounded sure of herself, "I didn't know that I could make any decisions about anything before we met Dr Phillips. I like that, Mom. It's scary too but I'm not doing this alone. I have you and Dad and I have a TEAM here... not just one doctor. And did you see the posters in the elevator? They have yoga and meditation sessions and they can help, right?"

Carol knew that her daughter was right. If she was going to be treated here, she would have the support of professionals like Angela and a whole team of health care providers. And in the websites that she had explored about cancer in young adults, they all talked about the need for young adults to be given choices about their treatment and for them to be involved in shared decision making with the doctors. But it was so hard to let go – of the responsibility of caring for their daughter and protecting her from harm.

"You're right, you're right…" she looked at Maddison, "This is the right place for you to have your treatment, and I am supportive of your choice, of course I am. Now let's tell Angela that we're ready to talk to Dr Phillips again. And let's get this started!"

Conclusion

Young adults, and even some older adolescents, newly diagnosed with cancer are capable of being involved in making decisions about their treatment. Shared decision-making where the professionals inform and guide the process, can help to reduce distress and may empower the person to continue to be involved in decisions as treatment progresses. Parents may find it challenging to let go of the control they want to have but ultimately, it is the young person who will truly experience the treatments and side effects.

Reflective Questions

After reading this story:

- What was the benefit for this family after asking for a second opinion?
- It is normal to feel guilt and/or a sense of responsibility when a child is diagnosed with cancer. What can you do to overcome these feelings that are ultimately not helpful?
- How can you encourage a young adult to be involved in making decisions about treatment? How does this impact on your role as primary care giver(s)?

4

CARING DURING TREATMENT

"I'VE NEVER SEEN ANYONE SO SICK;
I FEEL HELPLESS"

It seemed to Ashley and Peter that the past week had taken place over a lifetime. It started on Sunday when their 17-year old son Jonah had come down the stairs and Ashley noticed some bruises on his hands.

"Honey", she asked as she poured him some orange juice, "What have you done to yourself?"

Jonah glanced at his hands, first the left and then the right, and shrugged.

"Were you fighting with someone?" his dad joked.

"Uh, no..." Jonah did not seem particularly interested.

"Are you feeling okay, Jonah?" his mom persisted. "You've been sleeping a lot lately, like more than usual. Have you noticed any other changes?"

"Um, I'm not sure ... well, okay... there's this lump under my arm...."

Ashley looked at her husband, her face pale.

"Jonah, you need to come with me NOW and we're going to Urgent Care. Drink your juice and get dressed. I mean it. NOW!"

DOI: 10.4324/9781003242680-4

Peter looked at his wife, shocked by her outburst and what seemed like panic in her voice. Ashley was a medical librarian and had always joked that she should at least be given one year off medical school if she decided to make a career change.

"What is it? Ash, what are you thinking?" Peter sounded worried.

"I don't want to jump to conclusions, but those bruises and a lump may mean something really bad is happening..." Ashley had tears in her eyes that she brushed away. She could hear Jonah's footsteps coming down the stairs and she didn't want to worry him, at least not yet.

The three of them went to the Urgent Care clinic and that is when time sped up. A nurse practitioner asked Jonah a lot of questions, ordered some blood tests, and told him to go straight to the hospital emergency room. When they got there, they were whisked into an examination room and soon they were surrounded by a team of doctors and nurses and other people who were not introduced to them.

Jonah looked like someone had punched him in the stomach; Peter didn't look any better. Ashley had been taking notes as the doctors spoke, snatching a word or sentence here and there but in her gut, she knew. She had heard the acronym 'ALL' and she understood that all too well. Acute lymphocytic leukemia, a rapidly progressing type of blood and bone marrow cancer, that when treated had a good prognosis but she also knew that the treatment would be brutal for her son.

Within the hour he had a bone marrow aspiration; his parents sat in the waiting room while it was being done, holding hands but not talking to one another. They had sedated Jonah for the procedure, and he was sleepy when they were allowed to see him. He didn't look like their usual robust son; he was pale, and Ashley was reminded of how he looked when he was a baby, his eyelashes casting shadows over his cheeks. She wanted to put her arms around him and rock him as she used to. Peter stood silently on the other side of the bed, silent tears running down his cheeks. When Jonah's eyes opened, he turned around and blew his nose quietly.

Dr Katz advises:
The diagnosis of cancer, especially in an adolescent or young adult, comes as a shock to the family. It is not unusual for individuals of this age to ignore or not regard physical changes as a cause for concern.

Invincibility, immortality and immunity are hallmarks of people at this stage of life and they may not realize that any symptoms they have are suggestive of illness. It is not uncommon for people in this age group to experience a delay in diagnosis; cancer in adolescents and young adults is relatively rare and primary care providers may not suspect cancer when they present with symptoms.

Jonah was transferred to a special Adolescent and Young Adult unit on the seventh floor of the hospital. His parents barely noticed the brightly colored walls and the social area with a large TV, foosball table, and bean bags scattered on the floor. The room assigned to Jonah was large with a curtained off area where one of them could stay overnight if they wanted to.

"Can Sam spend the night too?" Jonah asked.

"Absolutely not!" Ashley's voice was too loud, and Peter whispered to her to lower the volume.

"But Mooommmmm", Jonah sounded like a four-year old, "Sam's my girlfriend and I need to see her…"

Now he had tears in his eyes. Ashley and Peter had not seen him cry since he was about ten years old. Last summer when he fell off his skateboard and broke his clavicle and cracked three ribs, he didn't cry, not even once. He didn't cry when their dog Mindy died, and she was his best friend since he was six years old. But now he cried, giant sobs that he tried to hide under his hands.

His father stepped closer to the bed and in a firm voice told both Jonah and his wife that they would discuss this another day. It was 1 pm, none of them had anything to eat since breakfast and even that had been cut short by their trip to Urgent Care.

"I'm going to go to the cafeteria to get us all something to eat. What do you want?"

Ashley couldn't even think about eating, but she recognized that she was beginning to feel nauseous and that she needed to put something in her stomach.

One of the nurses had entered the room and she interrupted them. "We have snacks in the kitchen just off the social area and you're welcome to take anything from there. And Jonah, you can call the kitchen downstairs and order anything you like from the menu on your side table. They make great French fries and you can ask them to put onion rings on a cheeseburger if you want."

"Why is there such unhealthy food available to patients?" Ashley sounded angry. She grabbed the menu and started reading. "And food can be ordered 24/7? That's just nuts!"

The nurse who had introduced herself as Brooks, spoke directly to Ashley.

"Many of our patients have no appetite because of their cancer or the treatments. We have found that having food that they want to eat whenever that is, does more good than harm, so our patients can eat what they want, at any time. And you know that these kids have a different inner clock so being able to get something yummy to eat after midnight is important".

Jonah smiled at his father who winked at him. There had been many nights over the past years when the two of them had bumped into each other in the dark kitchen. Those late-night snacks had led to deep conversations about baseball and girls and things that can only be said while eating cereal and cold lasagna.

Dr Katz advises:
   Specialized units for adolescents and young adults are created to provide age-appropriate care, including psychosocial support for patients. This may include availability of food around the clock, video games, TV and movies, as well as common areas where those who are well enough can gather. In addition, staff are trained to meet the needs of the patients, including having family members staying overnight as well as allowing friends to visit at any hour. The intent of these initiatives is to make the time that the young person spends in hospital as pleasant as possible, with due regard to their social and developmental needs.

The next day was a busy one for Jonah. He had numerous tests and imaging studies and later that afternoon, his hematologist, Dr Bradley, and his team met with Jonah and his family to talk about his treatment.

Ashley looked exhausted; she'd slept on the bed provided for visitors in Jonah's room but the constant overhead announcements, even through the night, disrupted her sleep. She had only taken time away from his bedside when Jonah had tests or when his girlfriend came to visit. She had finally relented and allowed Sam to spend time with Jonah in the evening when she showered and had dinner in the cafeteria, but she would not allow his girlfriend to sleep over.

Dr Bradley cleared his throat and began.

"We now have a much better picture of what is happening with Jonah and have a treatment plan that we want to start immediately. Jonah has acute lymphocytic leukemia, ALL, as we suspected and will need a stem cell transplant. His best bet for a stem cell donor is a member of your family and you should all be tested to see if you are a match. I see here that you have an older daughter, does she live here?"

Even though the diagnosis was not unexpected, Jonah's parents were in shock. The confirmation, the actual words spoken out loud felt like a physical blow. Jonah was silent, his eyes focused on something at the end of his bed.

"I understand that this is a shock to you all, but we need to get going on finding a stem cell donor for Jonah, and a family member is better than an unrelated donor".

"Jonah's sister, our daughter, well she lives in California…"

"We can work with our colleagues there to see if she is a match", the doctor responded.

"But she's 5 months pregnant!" Ashley once again was talking very loudly. The doctor seemed not to notice.

"Hmm, okay, I need to think about that. In the meantime, we would like to take some blood from the two of you and with luck, one or both of you will be a match. We do need to go ahead with the treatment for Josh in preparation for the stem cell transplant".

The doctor, a hematologist, went on to explain the phases of treatment that Jonah would undergo. Dr Bradley explained that these treatments were going to be hard on Jonah, but he would get through it.

Jonah had been silent as the doctor talked.

"Um, can I ask a question?" his voice was hesitant.

"Of course, Jonah", Dr Bradley replied, "I bet you have LOTS of questions!"

"How long am I going to be here?"

"That's a great question but unfortunately it has an 'it depends' answer", Dr Bradley had turned to look at Jonah, his back was now to Jonah's parents.

"Right after we stop talking, I am going to ask your parents to have a blood test to see if one of them can be a donor for you. I have my Fellow looking into whether your sister can be tested as well. We are going to start your chemotherapy this afternoon and you will have daily treatments until your transplant; this is called induction or conditioning therapy and it destroys the cancer cells as well as your bone marrow. Then we'll put the donor cells into your bloodstream, and they'll go to your bone marrow. After that, we have to wait and see. It'll take a couple of weeks for the stem cells from the transplant to start growing in your bone marrow. Once the stem cells have engrafted, our word for when the stem cells settle in the marrow and start growing, we have to monitor you carefully for some time. People your age do well and go home after a month or so. But I can't promise you anything, we have to see how you respond. Does that make sense?"

Jonah nodded; he was afraid that if he said anything he would start to cry, and he did NOT want to cry in front of the doctor.

"What can we expect in terms of side effects, Doc?" Peter's voice was a little shaky.

"The nurse will go through all of that with you", Dr Bradley replied as he moved towards the door, "I really do need to go and write the orders for Jonah's chemotherapy and also arrange for you two to have the blood tests. My apologies..."

And with that, he was gone, followed by the rest of his team who had not introduced themselves.

Ashley moved closer to her son and reached out to hug him, but Jonah shifted away from her.

"Honey, Ash...." Peter tried to take control of the situation that had nowhere to go but downhill, "Let's take a break here. I need coffee and Jonah needs some time alone, right son?"

Jonah looked up at his dad; the young man's eyes were full of tears and as one rolled down his cheek, he ducked his head and nodded.

"Peter, don't tell me what to do! Jonah needs us! Now more than ever..." Ashley's voice was strangled by the fear in her throat.

"Ash ... come on....." Peter was about to take her arm to get her out of the room, but she pulled away, almost falling against Jonah's bed.

"Mom!" Jonah's voice startled her, "Just go with Dad, PLEASE!"

Ashley was crying now, not making any attempt to stop. She pushed past her husband and walked quickly down the corridor and into the washroom down the hall. Brooks, the nurse they had met yesterday, followed her.

"Can I help, Ms ... um...Ashley?"

"Just go away, please... I need to be alone... just go! Please!"

Brooks left the washroom and almost bumped into Peter who was about to follow his wife.

"I don't mean to interfere..." Brooks spoke quietly but firmly, "But your wife just asked me to leave her alone. Maybe you need to just wait out here till she's ready to come out."

Dr Katz advises:

Reactions to bad news is different for everybody and may not reflect how people usually respond to changes. A life-threatening illness in child is the one of the worst things that can happen to parents, and it is difficult to anticipate how you will react. Some parents want to control what happens and become very protective. Depending on the age of the young person with cancer, this may be met with resistance. In this instance, Jonah at 17 years of age, is on the cusp of maturity and likely wants to make his own decisions; this can be difficult for parents to accept.

The family must, sooner rather than later, talk about how decisions will be made, who consents to treatment, who can receive medical information, and other issues related to treatment. This process may need to involve a social worker or other members of the cancer team as it is not always an easy process, especially for parents who may be reluctant to recognize their child's autonomy.

That afternoon Peter and Ashley gave blood samples to see if they could be donors for Jonah's stem cell transplant. They were told the results would be back in a couple of days and as the needle went into their vein, each said a silent prayer that they would be a match. They went back to Jonah's room, but he wasn't back yet. An older woman was waiting for them at the nurses' station.

"Hello, I'm Patricia, the social worker assigned to the AYA unit. But please call me Patty, everyone does!"

Peter and Ashley looked at each other; why did they need to see a social worker?

"I know what you're thinking", Patty said with a smile, "Why do we need to see a social worker?"

Jonah's parents looked a little embarrassed.

"Yeah, that's exactly what we were thinking", Ashley replied, "We're doing fine..."

She burst out crying again.

The social worker led them to a small room behind the nurses' station. Peter put his arm around his wife's shoulders but once again she pulled away. He hoped that Patty had not seen this; he was getting angry with her pulling away from him and it was embarrassing when this happened in front of other people.

One they were seated, Patty explained to them what her role was. Ashley had stopped sobbing and was now sniffing and wiping her nose on her sleeve. Patty passed her a box of tissues while she talked.

"My primary role here is to support the family and the young person as they go through the transplant process. Yes, the whole family. You are going to be challenged as you have never been challenged before, your son too in a different way. You may not feel like you need me now, but I know that nothing has prepared you for what is going to happen over the next weeks, and beyond".

She paused and waited for a response from the couple. But neither of them said anything.

"I am available to you, as a couple or as individuals, as Jonah goes through the transplant. I understand that you are both being tested to see if you can donate stem cells; it will be wonderful if you can. There are a lot of feelings associated with that too, and I am here to help either or both of you through this".

Peter cleared his throat. "I guess I would like to talk to you...."

Ashley's head shot up and she glared at him. How dare he involve this woman in their private life?

"Honey, I need to talk to someone! You don't have to if you don't want to, but I DO!"

"Are we done here?" Ashley's voice was clipped, and Peter looked away. "I need to be with my son so I'm leaving. You can do what you want, Peter, my only responsibility is to Jonah".

Peter didn't look at her as she got up and left the room; the door shut loudly behind her.

The social worker looked at him as he sighed, his eyes stared at his hands that rested on his thighs.

"It's hard, I know", she said softly, "Your wife's response is quite common".

"Is it?" Peter's voice was too loud in the small room, but Patty didn't seem to notice. "I thought we would face this together! But she's acting so weirdly…"

"Tell me how that feels, Peter", Patty replied.

And he did. He described how he couldn't seem to reach her, that she drew away from him when he tried to comfort her, and that she seemed distant and wouldn't talk to him about how she was feeling. And finally, in a quiet voice he told her that he was scared that their marriage was not going to survive.

Dr Katz advises:

In the time between diagnosis and the start of treatment, parents of an adolescent or young adult commonly experience a range of emotions such as fear, anxiety, distress, anger, and guilt to name just a few. They may grow closer together and support each other or they may retreat into themselves and become distanced. By not sharing their feelings with each other or a professional, they may experience an impact on their mental health such as depression and become even further isolated.

It may be difficult to share your fears with your partner/spouse. You may not want to increase their distress and so try to protect their feelings by not sharing your own suffering. This may not be productive; your partner may feel isolated and may suffer even more distress if they feel that they are facing things alone. Ultimately, this distancing is going to impact the young person with cancer who will sense the distance between their parents.

A social worker, psychologist, or family therapist can help you to address your feelings and to share with your partner/spouse how you are coping.

Jonah's induction chemotherapy started; the treatments was grueling, and he could barely get out of bed. On his better days he could take a few sips of apple juice or a spoonful of applesauce but on his worst days he was not able to even have a sip of water. His hair fell out in chunks and he didn't seem to notice. Brooks, his nurse, had warned them about the side effects but the reality was something else; Ashley left his room almost every hour to cry in the hallway. He was due to have full body radiation the next week and his mother could not even think about what that could do to his weakened body.

The only good news was that Peter was a match for Jonah and he would have the procedure to remove stem cells from his body when Jonah had completed the induction phase. Ashley had acted in an unexpected way when they were told that Peter was a match. She looked as if she was angry and Peter was shocked.

"Aren't you happy for us?" he asked one night on their drive home. Ashley was exhausted after a day when Jonah threw up, over and over again; the anti-nausea medications seemed to not work that day.

"Yes of course I am!" Ashely spat out the words, "But it should have been ME! I gave birth to him and I should be the one to save him!"

Peter was shocked. Was she jealous? He recognized that Jonah and his mother were close, always had been, but as Jonah grew older, his relationship with Peter had grown much closer too. But since Olivia, their older daughter, had moved to California, Ashley had doted on Jonah in a way that Peter thought was a little inappropriate for a young man of 17. As he thought about this, he realized that Sam, Jonah's girlfriend, had not been at the hospital.

"Ash, have you seen Sam lately? It's strange that she's not been around..."

"Hmmm" was the response.

"What does that mean? I thought we agreed that she could visit Jonah in the evening. Did you say something to her?"

Ashley sat silently, her eyes on the road.

"It all makes sense now!" Peter was getting angrier by the second and he drove into a parking lot, his hands shaking on the steering wheel. "You told her she couldn't visit him, didn't you? Why on earth would you do that? On top of everything else our son is going through, you decided to turn his girlfriend away! I... I can't believe that you would do something like that!"

"He's my son! My baby!" Ashley shouted at him. She hit the passenger side window with her fist. "He's my baby and I have to protect him! I have never seen him so sick! She has no right to visit him! What if she brings an infection into his room? That could kill him!"

Peter wanted her to stop yelling but he knew that if he told her to keep quiet, it would just make things worse. He tried to take some deep breaths to calm himself; he had never been so angry with her in the entire time they had been together.

"We are ALL risks to him, Ashley. You or I could expose him. That's why we wash our hands, put on those gowns and gloves before we enter his room. Oh, and the masks!"

He knew she was being irrational and so tried to get her to see where she was going wrong, but it was useless. Her reaction was emotional, and her feelings overrode any practical suggestions.

Dr Katz advises:

A parent is a parent for life and when one's child is in danger, the parent becomes protective, sometimes to extreme levels, and reacts like a bear protecting her/his cub. Rationality goes out the window and a more primal response takes over. The problem with this is that an adolescent or young adult has to gain autonomy and agency as they get older and they may revolt against the protective actions of a parent. They may feel as if they are being treated like an infant and this can impact negatively on their relationship with their parent(s). Keeping friends and partners away from the young person also removes an important aspect of social relationships and may cause or increase depression.

While the risk of infection is a concern for someone who is being treated with chemotherapy, especially in high doses such as those given before a stem cell transplant, the cancer care team is aware of this and provides gowns, masks and gloves to visitors and monitors the patient for any signs of infection. Hand washing is essential for all staff and visitors interacting with the patient and certain foods (for example vegetable sprouts, raw or undercooked meat) are not allowed.

Finally, the day of the transplant arrived. Jonah was at his sickest. He had lost weight, his veins were visible, blue streaks that meandered like streams under his pale skin. He barely acknowledged his parents who stood excitedly at his bedside, their eyes glued to the bag of red liquid that dripped Peter's stem cells into their child's body. The procedure was almost a let-down; the cells went in, but nothing changed. Jonah lay there, his eyes fluttering under his eyelids, just as they had done when he was a baby. But there was no demanding cry of "Mamma, Mamma" as was usual when he woke from his nap. He was so still, and Ashley felt like her heart was cracking in her chest. It was an actual physical pain and she could bear it no longer. She ran from the room, almost knocking Patty the social worker into the wall.

"Is she okay?" Patty whispered to Peter who just shrugged. He was still looking at the IV tubing that had dripped his cells into Jonah.

"I don't know what happened … she's been like this for a while. I wish she would talk to you, she's really not herself…"

"I'll try again, Peter", the social worker's voice was soft, and he smiled at her.

"Isn't this amazing, Patty? Just look, part of MY body went into Jonah's and this may…" his voice cracked, "This may be the start of hope for him…"

Patty put her hand on his arm.

"Sure is, and for you too, Peter. We should maybe talk about YOUR feelings with all this. Being a donor for a loved one is not always straight forward. It has weight and implications for you and your family for the rest of your lives".

Dr Katz advises:

Being a stem cell donor for a loved one is life altering for the donor as well as the recipient. Besides the physical impact of donating the cells (pain, bruising, fatigue) there are emotional ones as well. Donors may be concerned that their donation won't 'take' (engraft) because they did or didn't do something. If the transplant of their cells does not help the patient, they may feel guilty. There are multiple factors that determine the outcome of the stem cell transplant, and there is nothing that the donor can do to ensure success.

There are also implications for family members who would like to donate their stem cells but are not a good match. This can cause grief, anger and frustration that they were not 'chosen'. They may resent the family member who was able to donate, and this can cause conflict.

Jonah's recovery was slow, just as the hematologist had warned. But every day he gained a little; he was soon able to go to the washroom in his room by himself. He was given a walker but preferred to hold onto the furniture and walls. "I am NOT an old man!" was his response to Brooks, his nurse, when she suggested that using the walker was safer. What really cheered him up was when Sam came to visit. They were really careful about this because his mom had insisted that Sam could only visit when she was there. This was not fun for either of them, so they figured out a plan; Sam would come first thing in the morning on her way to class when neither of his parents was around. Ashley had stopped sleeping at the hospital after his transplant; the hourly checks by the night nurses were also disruptive to her sleep. So, between 6 am and 8 am, Sam and Jonah were alone and could do what they wanted.

About three weeks after his transplant, Jonah was walking in the hallway, assisted by Sam who had her arm around his waist. Sam suddenly stopped and Jonah almost fell.

"Oh shit", she whispered, "Jonah, it's your Mom! She's going to kill me!"

"Huh??" Jonah looked up and there she was, his mother was coming towards them and the look on her face was scary.

"Jonah! What is SHE doing here? And what are you doing out of your room?"

She turned to glare at Sam.

"You know you're not supposed to be here! Has this been happening every day? You need to leave RIGHT NOW!"

Brooks and the other nurses heard this exchange. Brooks was there within seconds and ushered them into the small office where Patty usually talked to families.

Ashley turned on Brooks as soon as the door closed behind them.

"Did YOU know about this, Brooks? How could you let this happen? It's not safe! What if she makes him sick? What else has been happening behind my back?"

Brooks waited until Ashley took a breath.

"Ashley, I did know about this. And I think that Sam is an important part of Jonah's recovery".

Ashley started to interrupt.

"Please, let me finish. I understand that this is very difficult for you and I also know that you are angry that your wishes were not followed. But Jonah is 17, he is not a baby. And he must be allowed to have some choices in this. I want you to have a chat with Patty and yes, I know you don't want to..."

Brook's voice was firm.

"Patty is on her way. Let's let Jonah and Sam go back to his room and I'll get you some water while we wait." She looked at Jonah and his girl-friend, "Go on, you two, off you go!"

Patty arrived a minute later. She was out of breath and looked like she needed some water too.

"Thanks, Brooks. I'll take it from here. Good morning Ashley! Or perhaps I should ask how your morning has been?"

As the door to the office closed, Ashely started to talk; she did not stop for the next 20 minutes. Patty did not have to ask her anything, it all spilled out and over. Ashley described being terrified that her darling boy would die. She was hurt and jealous that she was not a match. Peter seemed disconnected from her and did not seem to be as scared as she was. She felt helpless and now that he had the transplant, any hope that she thought that would bring had been replaced by fear that it would not take. And he might die.

Patty sat and listened. She had heard similar stories from other parents, and she knew that Ashley needed to talk until she had no words left. Eventually Ashley stopped and gave a big sigh. Patty validated her feelings, telling her that what she felt was universal for parents of a sick child, no matter how old. But she also told Ashley that Jonah was not a child anymore; he was a young man who had come through the worst experience of his life, and he needed to have as normal a life now as he possibly could.

"I know that, Patty! But I am so scared. Every moment of every day. It's the last thing I think of at night as I go to sleep and the first thing when I wake up in the morning. And I am SO mad that Sam is here when I distinctly told them that she could only visit when I was here!"

"Why are you so angry about Sam being here this morning?" Patty asked gently, "Is it the fact that they were going against your wishes or that Sam was here in the first place?"

"I don't know ... maybe it's that she's here when I'm not and I'm scared that she'll bring in something that will make him sick...Does she even follow the rules about protecting him?"

"Why don't we ask Brooks about that? She'll know if Sam has been following the rules and wearing all the protective gear. But let's talk about your feelings about Sam and Jonah's relationship because I think that's at the root of your reaction today".

Dr Katz advises:

It can be difficult for parents to accept another important person in their child's life and this is even harder when they are in 'protection mode'. But as children grow older, establishing romantic and sexual relationships are important developmental milestones. As children grow up, a negotiation has to take place with their parent(s) as all their roles change. The parent is no longer the center of the young person's life and others will become the love object, as much as that hurts the parent who has loved and focused on the wellbeing of their child from infancy. Instead of trying to sabotage the relationship, it would be wiser to accept the girl- or boy-friend as an ally, someone who can help the parents take care of their adolescent or young adult child.

Ultimately, all that the parents of a young person with cancer can do is to love their child. The loss of control that comes with a cancer diagnosis and the ensuing treatment is out of their control. Being over-protective and not allowing their child to have autonomy or agency is confusing for the young person and can lead to distancing and rebellion.

Ashley nodded as Patty talked. Part of her knew she was out of control and that her reaction to seeing Sam that morning was exaggerated. She agreed to talk to Jonah and Sam about her worries and she even volunteered that she owed them an apology.

Patty smiled as she heard that; it was unexpected but absolutely the right thing for Ashley to do. Even a Mamma bear needs to share the load of caring for her cub sometimes.

Conclusion

A life-threatening illness in a child, not matter how young or old, is a life-changing experience for parents. The loss of control, fear of their child not surviving the treatments, and disruption of the expected order of things, all contribute to personal and couple functioning. Instead of supporting each other, parents may fight each other, despite the strong bonds that once held them together. When an adolescent or young adult has a partner, this may cause additional problems as one or both parents may be overprotective of their child, attempting to sabotage or end the relationship. These reactions often result in poor outcomes for the person with cancer and their relationship with their parents.

Reflective Questions

After reading this story:

- How can you as a parent avoid being overprotective when your adolescent or young adult child is diagnosed and treated for cancer?
- What strategies can you use to give up control of things you have no control over and yet find some things that you can control?
- How have you dealt with the boy- or girlfriend of your child? What advice would you give to another parent in a similar situation?

5

LIVING WITH CANCER

"WHO CAN HELP US AT THIS TIME"?

Julie, aged 34 years and her husband Nate, 36, have a 12-month old baby named Jack. Julie and Nate have been married for four years. Jack was a very much wanted baby, conceived after two years of trying to get pregnant. They were about to start fertility treatments when Julie found out she was pregnant and they decided to put the money they were going to spend on getting pregnant into renovating their garage into a 'granny suite'. Nate's mother Adele lived about 1,000 miles away and after her husband and Nate's father died suddenly of a heart attack, she was lonely and wanted to visit them often. Once Jack was born, her frequent visits had turned into two- and three-month stays; Julie was really glad that they now had a space for her, even if it was only 25 steps from their back door. Julie's parents, Brian and Cheryl, lived a five-minute car ride away and visited only when invited.

Julie found a lump in her left breast when Jack was nine months old. She was not that concerned as one of the other moms in the Baby and Me yoga class she attended had told the group that she had found a lump, but it was mastitis, and it went away after she took antibiotics. But Julie had

DOI: 10.4324/9781003242680-5

none of the other symptoms of mastitis and the lump did not go away. It was not painful, but it was still there two months later. She reported this to her primary care provider who ordered a mammogram and then an MRI and finally, Julie had a biopsy. She had breast cancer and it was the 'bad one', a triple negative breast cancer that is often aggressive and not responsive to medications that prevent a recurrence in the future. Within weeks she had a mastectomy and was devastated to learn that she had to have chemotherapy as well; she could no longer breastfeed Jack and in some ways, this felt worse than having cancer.

Nate took a leave from his work as an architect; Julie had to switch her maternity leave to a medical leave. Nate's mom Adele flew back to live with them, even though they hadn't asked her to. Julie's parents were helpful; Cheryl helped Julie to bathe, cooked her favorite foods, and helped Nate with Jack's bath time. Brian was always willing to go to the grocery store for supplies and he would swing Jack on the baby swing for as long as the child wanted.

Julie did not always get on well with her mother-in-law; it was fine when her husband John was alive, but now she was demanding of Nate's attention and this annoyed Julie. While Julie was recovering from the surgery, Adele would come over multiple times during the day, mostly uninvited. If Julie's parents were there, she would sit and watch TV and not offer to help with anything. She didn't approve of Julie continuing to breastfeed Jack from her remaining breast, and once when Julie was taking a nap, she gave Jack a bottle of water because he was "dying of thirst". Julie was furious with her; she didn't want Jack taking a bottle. She wanted to breastfeed for as long as possible, cherishing every quiet moment with him as he nursed, his big brown eyes staring into hers until his eyelids gave in to sleep.

Dr Katz advises:
Relationships with family members can be stressed by a cancer diagnosis and the resultant need for care and support. People generally like to help and want to feel needed, but this can be a delicate situation. In-laws may find that their attempts to 'help' are unwanted, and this leads to hurt feelings and even conflict. Views on child-rearing are often a flashpoint for arguments as seen when Julie's mother-in-law

gives baby Jack a bottle. For Julie this is unacceptable even if it was done with good intent. Julie is mourning the loss of her ability to breastfeed in the future and this loss further traumatizes her after the cancer diagnosis and what this means for their future.

Nate had to talk to his mother after this. He tried to be gentle with her, but she reacted to his words with tears and threats to go back to her home because she wasn't wanted by him. Nate was used to this kind of reaction from her; she had been doing it his whole life and he had always given her what she wanted. But now he had a wife who was sick, and a baby who needed his mother.

"Mom", he tried to keep his voice under control, "We are very appreciative of your help, really we are. But you have to realize that Julie is Jack's mother and what she says, goes. No bottles, not until Julie starts chemo. No, don't interrupt me, please"!

But Adele did just that. "He has to get used to bottles so what's the harm with a little water? He was gasping from thirst! I should know what that looks like. And YOU were bottle-fed until you were three…"

Nate's anger spilled over; he was scared about Julie's cancer and their future, and his mother was not helping with that old story about him and bottles.

"I asked you not to interrupt and there you went! It's always like this with you! You always know better! It's your way or the highway! And frankly, the next time you threaten to go home, I won't try to prevent you from doing just that!"

He walked away without looking at her. He knew she was crying again, and this time he had to avoid her emotional manipulation. His first responsibility was to Julie and Jack. Why could Adele not see how stressed he was?

Dr Katz advises:

In times of stress, conversations about sensitive topics can quickly become arguments that may hurt feelings and change relationships. When a parent and a grown child are forced to live in close quarters because of illness, an addition to the family, or other stressors, the parent may fall back into old ways of treating their now adult child. And the reverse is true as well! The adult child may revert to behaviors from their early years (drinking out of the juice container in front of the fridge?).

Trying to establish boundaries for help and support can feel like rejection to the parent, even though it is intended to protect a spouse/partner who did not grow up with that parent. Hurt feelings can turn into defensiveness and threats. This is difficult territory and when things feel like they are dissolving into chaos, that is the time to step away, take a few deep breaths, and return to the initial conversation when everyone has calmed down. No good will come from continuing to argue or explain when harsh words are said.

Nate went back into the house, his shoulders lowered as if carrying a heavy weight.

"That obviously didn't go well", Julie recognized the signs in her husband after he had talked to his mother. It had happened before; just before their wedding Adele had insisted on planning the seating arrangements for the reception even though Julie and Nate didn't want assigned seating. It hadn't ended well; she threatened to leave before the wedding and it was only when her husband, Nate's kind and gentle father John, took her aside and spoke to her for 20 minutes, his voice louder than Julie had ever heard, that she relented. Adele didn't leave but she gave them both the silent treatment, even up to the wedding ceremony in Julie's parents' garden. Julie was relieved that Adele didn't talk to either of them, the absence of her 'advice' made the day go smoother.

"I don't know why it also goes south whenever I try to talk to her", Nate's anger flared again. "She does the same thing, over and over. She threatens to leave and tells me how much she misses my Dad and on and on…. But this time I didn't fold. I walked away but now I feel so guilty…"

He left out the part where his mother had defended herself about the bottle she gave to Jack. He really didn't want to upset Julie and that would certainly upset her. She was starting chemotherapy in just a few days; he knew she was anxious, and he was too. Their life was about to change even more, and there were times when he wanted it all to be just a nightmare. But it was their reality now, and he hoped he could get through the next nine months without falling apart himself.

Julie's parents returned to the house later that afternoon; they had made Julie's favorite chicken pot pie and had a couple of bottles of craft beer for Nate. Jack was in his highchair and he shouted with delight when he saw them. Julie's mother hugged her and immediately started cleaning the kitchen counter where Nate had prepared Jack's early dinner.

"Please stop that, Mom", Julie hated to feel so helpless, but her chest was still painful after her mastectomy and her left arm was weak after hardly being used since the surgery. She had been told to see a physiotherapist to start rehabilitation on that arm, but where did she have time? Taking care of Jack, even with her parents' and Nate's help, meant she had little time for herself.

"Let's go for a walk, Nate", Brian said to his son-in-law.

He could see the strain on the young man's face, and he wanted to give Julie and her mother time to talk. Nate looked at Julie, waiting for permission to leave her.

"Go!" Julie waved him off. "I want to talk to my mom. Remember to check for mail on your way back…"

Nate put on his baseball cap, waved goodbye to Jack who was throwing peas, one by one, onto the floor. The little guy looked so happy, he thought, if only we could keep it like this…

"How are you holding up, honey?" Cheryl ran her hand over her daughter's hair. Her heart ached as she thought about that beautiful hair falling out as she knew it would during chemotherapy.

"Oh mom", Julie tried not to cry, but she too was thinking about her hair, "I don't know how I'm going to cope! I am dreading the chemotherapy. Last night I was thinking about refusing it, or maybe asking if I can delay it…. I don't want to stop breastfeeding. Jack's still small and he needs my milk!! I hate this, all of this! I know I shouldn't ask why this happened to me, but why did it?"

The tears ran down her cheeks and to Cheryl, she looked like the little girl who got frustrated at the slightest failure to accomplish something.

"Oh, honey…." Cheryl started to comfort her, "You've done so well breastfeeding for this long … I stopped when you were…"

"Mom! I don't need you to try to make me feel better! Nothing you say will make this better, nothing!"

Dr Katz advises:

Parents often try to explain and rationalize in an attempt to comfort, but often that isn't what is needed. Just listening and letting the other person vent is usually what is wanted. Advice can be experienced as a lecture and who likes to be lectured to? And advice is not the same as support, and support is one of the most important things a parent can provide to their child with cancer, and to their partner too.

There are different types of support: tangible, informational, and emotional. Tangible support, in the form of helping with household or childcare tasks, is often the most appreciated as couples dealing with cancer face challenges including fatigue, both physical and emotional. Informational support is usually provided by health care providers or knowledgeable friends and family, and people searching for information on the internet. Emotional support is shown by just being present and listening. Parents may feel that they must DO something; hearing the suffering of a child, even one who has children of their own, is not easy. But the person who is struggling may not want answers, just someone to hear them and validate what they are going through.

Julie started chemotherapy on with a 'one week on, three weeks off' schedule. The week that she had treatments were rough; she slept most of the time she was home and Jack had started to say "Shhh, shhhh" when he passed her room on his way to bed. Nate was being pressured to go back to work and he was considering quitting his job and going solo once Julie was better. His father-in-law reminded him that he would lose his insurance coverage, and so he arranged to go back every month for the three weeks that Julie was recovering from chemotherapy; he agreed to take a cut in his salary so that he could be home the week Julie had her treatments.

Cheryl and Brian came to the house every day to play with Jack and help Julie. They took great care of their grandson and rejoiced in each milestone he achieved. On the weeks that Julie didn't have chemotherapy, she would sit on the deck and watch as her father taught 16-month old Jack how to throw a ball. The boy chuckled when he managed to pick up the bright red ball and heave it toward his beloved Papa, his name for Brian. Adele had been helping too; she mostly stayed in the granny suite when Cheryl and Brian were there, despite their repeated invitations to join them for coffee or in the yard when they were out-side with Jack. She helped with the laundry and vacuuming, chores that Nate usually did. Julie thought that she only did things that her son was supposed to do, but she knew this was spiteful and didn't say anything to Nate.

Nate was grateful for the help from his in-laws and his mother, but he was beginning to feel useless. Cheryl took care of Julie so well; she bathed her daughter when Julie was too sick or weak, she made bland foods that Julie loved as a child – rice pudding, custard and jelly, and homemade macaroni and cheese. Nate found that completing tasks at work was taking much longer than it did before. He was distracted and made some rookie mistakes while drafting plans for a client who wanted to work only with him. Nate appreciated the client's support and so he stayed late at work so that he could meet the deadline for the architec-tural plans. He got home exhausted, often to find that Cheryl had put Jack to sleep before Nate could see him. His father-in-law was always ready to do the weekly shopping and sometimes he bought candy and other treats for Jack that he and Julie had agreed their toddler should not be having. But he was too tired to argue and so just ignored that. And then there was his mother who demanded that he spend time with her in the evenings. Once or twice he had fallen asleep as she went on and on with her complaints about her various aches and pains.

Dr Katz advises:
    Help from parents and others can be overwhelming despite how grateful a partner/spouse may be. Feeling not needed as others step in to take care of your partner can exacerbate your distress and/or depression. Family relationships can be difficult; family caregivers are themselves reacting to their adult child's illness and may feel power-less to change what has happened and so they become protective, sometimes to the exclusion of the partner. The person with cancer may welcome the attention of his/her parent(s) as a retreat into childhood patterns of behavior may bring comfort.

It is important to set boundaries before problems occur. The survivor's partner should be involved in making decisions about who is responsible for what; they are the one who may need as much support as the person with cancer. Parents and other family members are not going to do things exactly as you and your partner might, but that is perhaps a sacrifice that you may be prepared to make to alleviate some of your stress. A list of who does what and when, posted on the fridge, will provide clear guidelines for everyone.

The goal of parents or other family members should be to help and support you and your partner; the way this plays out can be welcome or a source of stress. Open and honest communication about what both you and your partner need is key to making this work.

Nine months is a long time but finally Julie's chemotherapy treatments ended. She was weak and had lost all her hair, but she was now on the other side of treatment and she started to recover slowly. Her parents were still taking care of Jack most of the time; her mother-in-law had left three months before and that was a relief to everyone, including Nate. It was only after she was gone that he was able to relax. Her constant demands for his attention had been more draining than he had realized and now he could focus solely on Julie and Jack, who at almost two years, was a busy little boy who mumbled to himself and was clear in what he wanted and he mostly wanted things NOW!

Nate had gone back to work full time and the extra income was welcome. He was also making an effort to come home before Jack went to bed; he and Julie would sit and watch him in the bathtub, his hair full of bubbles as he splashed and shouted at them to "Look Dadda! Look Mamma!". After they read him a story, they had time to themselves and one evening, Julie suggested to Nate that it was time he went out with his friends. He had not seen any of his friends for months, and the truth was he missed them. But on the other hand, none of them had contacted him recently. They didn't ask how Julie was doing or if he could do with support. He had bumped into two of them at their local coffee shop and they didn't ask him to join them at their table. He was annoyed but he had little time to stew over the incident; he had bigger problems at the time and so just let it go. He didn't tell Julie any of this; she would just get angry at them and she didn't need to waste her energy on them.

Julie insisted that he go out with them for a couple of beers. He agreed reluctantly and called Joe, the informal organizer of the group. They were meeting to watch a baseball game two nights later and Nate said he would meet them at the bar. The night did not go well. They welcomed him with their usual jokes and settled in to watch the game. Nate was never a huge baseball fan, he preferred hockey and football in the winter, and he felt left out of the conversation. In between innings they joked around about their wives and Nate became even more irritated. Firstly, he didn't think joking around about one's wife was appropriate, but secondly, not one of them asked how Julie was doing. They all knew she had been sick, and they should have known that he was stressed, but not a word was said. After 45 minutes he got up and headed for the exit.

"Why are you leaving, guy? Don't be like that! The game is just getting interesting!" Their voices were too loud and other people at the bar were looking at them.

"I gotta go, that's all!" mumbled Nate.

He fumed the whole way home. Julie was surprised that he was back so early. She could see how angry he was, and he told her what had happened.

"Yeah…. I hear you. Did you notice that MY friends were also MIA for the most part?"

Nate hadn't really noticed the absence of her friends, some of whom were married to his friends.

"They mostly came in the beginning, when I first started chemotherapy. My mom told them that the week of treatment I was not feeling well enough for visitors, so they came when I was off treatment those three weeks. You were at work and I guess I didn't tell you. They brought their kids with them and honestly, I found the noise too much. And the worst part of it was that they just sat around, and my poor Mom had to make coffee and tea and serve them like it was some kind of tea party!"

Nate couldn't help it, he started to laugh and Julie joined him. What a bunch of immature losers their friends were!

Dr Katz advises:

The support of friends is important when you someone is dealing with any kind of serious health issue, but the intensity of their support often wanes as the months of treatment go by. What is experienced as a shock and an emergency at the time of diagnosis is difficult to sustain and so they may stop visiting or calling. Some say that this is the time when people realize who their real friends are, but that is not 100% accurate. Friends may have their own history of someone in their family getting sick and perhaps even dying. This will influence how they are able to interact with a friend who is ill.

Everyone is busy with their own lives; this is not an excuse for not supporting or helping the family in times of need, but it is a reality. Friends will often say "How can I help you"? and this places the onus on the person with cancer or their caregiver(s) to tell them what is needed. It is much more supportive for visitors to DO something when they come to visit; they can load or unload the dishwasher, do a load of laundry, pick up the kids' toys etc. But that also means that they should be allowed to do this!

Bringing food to the house is also helpful but if this is not organized well, there will be too many dinners one week and not enough the other weeks. A website such as CareCalendar (https://www.carecalendar.org) can be helpful in organizing help and avoiding overlaps.

Julie regained energy as the months went by. On the one-year anniversary of her diagnosis her parents prepared a small party to celebrate this milestone. Julie was dreading this; the year that had passed had left her anxious and afraid. As Jack grew, he became more and more fun, but she had missed so much of his development. He sometimes called for her mother when he needed something, and this hurt Julie more than she could say. Of course, she had not said anything to Cheryl, who had been more of a mother to Jack for the past year than she had. Nate also felt left out; they talked about this one night and sharing their feelings felt good. Nate told her that as much as he was grateful for all their help, and they had helped a LOT, he wanted them to spend less time at the house. Julie did not know what to do with this information; she depended so much on her mom, and to tell them that they were no longer needed felt like a betrayal. She stayed silent as she thought about how she could talk to them about this. Nate seemed to take her silence as agreement. He yawned, kissed her on the top of head, and went to bed.

The next morning Julie called her primary care provider and asked for a referral to a counsellor. She had not slept much the night before as she tried to figure out how to ask her parents to stay away more without hurting their feelings. She knew that she was not going to be able to do this without offending someone, and she really didn't want to hurt her parents, or Nate. It could not have been easy for him this past year, she thought. Despite getting on well with his in-laws, their almost constant presence had an impact on him too. He had to be fully dressed at all times, and Cheryl did tend to take over so even if he wanted to do laundry or make a meal, she stepped in and did it herself. Julie knew she had to talk to someone about how to talk to her parents...

Dr Katz advises:
There is a delicate balance when providing support and care to a loved one: when to continue at the level you did when they were sick and when to step back when they are on their way to resuming their usual life. It feels good to be needed and to help, especially when the person who is sick is a beloved adult child. It is easy to revert to the parent you used to be when they were small, where you attended to their every need and made them feel safe. But when your child is an adult, and they have a life partner of their own, you run the risk of overstepping a boundary that may be invisible and alienating the partner. Everyone has fragile feelings at times like these, and offence and misunderstandings happen easily.

Open and honest communication at multiple times over the course of your caregiving is important. This helps to make expectations clear and offers opportunities to reflect on what needs to be done and by whom. As your family member recovers from the intensity of treatment, it is reasonable to expect family caregivers to take some steps away from caregiving to allow everyone to re-establish their roles and identity as they did in the 'before' times

Julie was able to make an appointment with a counselor for the next week. She was a bit nervous talking to someone about such personal issues, but she knew she needed to do this. Nate and her mother were now barely talking to each other. Cheryl arrived at the house after Nate had left for work and made sure that she left before he came home. Julie asked her mother if Nate had done something to offend her and her mother insisted that everything was fine between them. Nate said the same thing about his relationship with her mother – but it was obvious that almost nothing was right between them!

The counsellor's office was located close to the hospital where Julie had her mastectomy. She glanced over at the large glass covered building as she drove past, and shivered. It all came back to her; walking into the hospital the morning of her surgery and going home the next day with the bulky dressing covering the left side of her chest and under her arm. In retrospect, that was the easy part. The recovery was much more painful than she anticipated. But that was in the past, she reminded herself as she parked her car in the lot behind the counselor's office.

The counselor's name was Dr Bennett. She was about the same age as Julie, with light brown hair tied in a messy bun on top of her head, and tortoise shell glasses that covered almost the entire top of her face. She welcomed Julie into her office that was decorated in shades of grey and blue.

"Have a seat on the couch, Julie. And if you want to take off your shoes, that's fine with me. I find that bare feet tend to ground us, don't they?"

Julie had no idea what to she was supposed to do but she took off her shoes and placed her bare feet on the soft rug.

"So how can I help you today?" Dr Bennett asked.

"Um, well I guess I called when I was really frustrated one day and that's when I called…"

"Okay, can you tell me a little more about WHY you were frustrated?"

Dr Bennett looked at Julie with expectation. This was not unusual for clients to forget why they needed to see her even though they sounded desperate when they called for an appointment.

"Okay … here goes…" Julie took in a deep breath and told the psychologist everything. She talked uninterrupted for almost ten minutes as Dr Bennett listened, nodding her head every now and then.

"You've been through a LOT", she said, "But can you tell me what three things are most bothersome to you at the present time?"

"Hmmm…" Julie needed to think for a moment, "I think I need to talk about the relationship we have with my parents. They've been amazing through my treatment, but I'm feeling better now and they… well it's mostly my mom ... she can't let go! She's great with Jack, our 2-year old, and I don't know what I would have done if she hadn't been here to help, but she needs to step back! We need to get our family back, Nate and I do, but how can I tell her that? It will hurt her, and I don't want to do that after all she's done for us..."

Dr Bennett nodded her head. She had seen this situation before, and it was a challenging one.

"What else can you tell me? How about starting by telling me about your parents, about Nate, and how things were before you got cancer?"

Julie told her everything; she adored her parents, and they her. She was an only child and the three of them had always been close. She could tell them anything, about school friends and boyfriends, and they always listened and never judged her, at least they never voiced any judgement to her. When she met Nate, they immediately welcomed him into their threesome. Nate's relationship with his own mother was not an easy one, and the unconditional affection that Cheryl had shown to him drew him ever closer into their family. But now there was tension; Nate had told Julie that he felt useless and resented how fully Cheryl had inserted herself into their daily life. But he went to work every day and Julie needed her mom to help with Jack. She felt caught in the middle and she didn't know how to fix this.

"It's not a good feeling, I know" Dr Bennett's voice was calm. "I do have some suggestions that might help..."

Dr Katz advises:

Despite the success of treatment, parents will continue to worry about their adult child's health and even though they may not talk about it, their anxiety may be overwhelming. In response they continue to behave just as they did in the crisis of treatment. Perhaps in some way they think that if they are constantly vigilant, nothing bad will happen. This is not reality of course, but feelings often don't reflect reality!

Being able to help and support the family also makes parents feel good; when someone feels helpless in a situation, being active in helping with childcare and household chores may decrease these feelings of helplessness. And of course, there is the joy in spending time with a grandchild. But there needs to be a balance and negotiating that balance can be a daunting task.

As in any difficult conversation, starting with 'I' statements can be useful: "I feel overwhelmed when you take over from me in caring for our child/doing the laundry now that I feel better". When you start with 'You do this...' the other person will automatically feel defensive and may argue with you.

Tell the person how their actions make you feel: "I feel like a child when you take over doing things that I can do now that I am back to my usual energy level".

It is important to ask them to act in a way that makes the situation better for you: "I would love for you to continue seeing [name of child] but it needs to be when it is good for us, and that is not all the time".

Then you can describe the benefits from making this change: "If you spend three afternoons a week with [name of child], I can go to my yoga class and you will have him/her all to yourself".

Julie was so pleased that she had met with the counselor. The appointment had ended with Julie receiving a list of statements that she could use to start the conversation with her parents. She had also made an appointment for both Nate and her to talk to Dr Bennett; their relationship had changed during her treatment and there were tensions and unspoken feelings that needed to be aired.

Conclusion

The relationship between parents, an adult child with cancer and their partner is often a close one, and after a diagnosis of cancer, the relationship may become even closer. There is a two-way benefit for support and practical help during this time; parents may be able to help, and this brings them satisfaction. The couple dealing with the cancer will usually appreciate the help from people that they love and trust. But there also needs to be boundaries and time limits set for this help. If not, resentment and conflict may occur that can affect the relationship permanently. Recovery from cancer is not just a physical experience, it is an emotional and relational one as well. Many survivors experience great personal growth from going through the diagnosis, treatment, and recovery; if there is anything positive to say about this, this personal growth is one.

Reflective Questions

After reading this story:

- How and when should boundaries for involvement with a sick adult child be set?
- If you are the partner of someone with cancer, what could you do to accept help and avoid resentment when others step in to help?
- What are signs that say the relationship with your child's partner/spouse and you is not going well and how can these be addressed in a positive way?
- What are some ways that you as the parent of a sick adult child can include activities that help with your own anxiety and distress?

6

THE AFTERMATH

"I WANT TO HAVE A NORMAL A LIFE"!

Todd Kohler is 17-years old and is starting his senior year in high school. He's one of the popular guys; six feet tall with the build of an athlete. He has always dressed like a model for Gap with pressed jeans or chinos, and clean t-shirts and sneakers. His friends tease him about this, but he takes their words in stride and maintains his standards. His black hair is also always clean and well groomed, his long eyelashes the envy of the girls in his class. Todd loves all sports, but football is his life. He expects to be captain of his high school football team in his senior year and has hopes of a college scholarship.

As close as he is with his group of friends and teammates, there is something that he has never told anyone. Last year he was diagnosed with testicular cancer. One day in the shower he noticed that one of his testicles was larger than the other. He wasn't sure what to do about it, and he was too embarrassed to tell his mother. At the time his father Vince was deployed to Afghanistan for the third time. Vince is a Marine and has not been around much for years. This was difficult for Todd to understand when he was younger, but his father's service and status as a

DOI: 10.4324/9781003242680-6

Marine is now a source of great pride. A wall in his bedroom is covered in photos of his father from all his deployments overseas as well as the official photo with the American flag behind him, his square jaw and blue eyes that Todd inherited making him look like a superhero.

It was late Fall when Todd noticed the difference in the size of his testicles; he had no pain so he just left it, hoping it would change with time. But it didn't. His dad came home on leave for Christmas and one day Todd told him what he had found. His dad didn't panic and said he'd ask Todd's mom, Michelle, to make an appointment with the pediatrician.

"Oh Dad! Must she do it? Can't I call Dr … what's his name?" Todd had not seen the pediatrician for three years at least. When his dad was away, his mom was distracted most of the time. She was a teacher at the local elementary school and she also taught some kids after school for a little extra money. Todd knew the he needed to see a doctor, but he was embarrassed.

"Dad, can't you call? Please? I don't want Mom to know…."

"Man up, Todd!" Vince used his Marine voice, "You're almost 18 and it's time you started to act like it! Firstly, you shouldn't be hiding things from your mother. And secondly, you can call Dr … um, I forget his name…I'll ask your Mom… and I'll try to not tell her why…"

Todd smiled; his father couldn't remember the doctor's name either!

After Todd called the pediatrician's office, things moved fast. He went to the appointment with his dad on a Thursday while his mother was at school and the following Monday he saw another doctor who did an ultrasound. They went back to the pediatrician at the end of the week, this time with his mother as well.

The pediatrician's face was serious when he entered the examination room; Todd and his parents were sitting silently, his parents on the only two chairs and Todd on the examination table.

"I wish I didn't have to tell you this, but Todd, you have testicular cancer".

Todd was calm as the pediatrician said these words. He looked at his parents; Todd's mother, gasped, her face white and her eyes wide. His father did not seem to react, except for a muscle on the side of his face, contracting and relaxing.

"How? Why? Now what?" Todd's mother had started to cry.

"Is it my fault, Doc?" Todd's father spoke too loudly. "I've been deployed three times. I've been exposed to all sorts of stuff…. Heavy metals, weird germs and things…."

"I know this is hard to hear, Mr and Mrs Kohler". The doctor's voice suggested that he had been in this situation before. "We still have to do another couple of tests and then Todd will need to see a specialist. We really don't have a good sense of why this happens to young men like Todd. There is nothing you have done that might have caused this. Right now I need to talk to Todd about some things. Todd, do you want your parents to leave?"

"Um, I don't know … do they have to"?

"No, they can stay if you wish. You're 17, almost 18, and you have the ability to make some choices regarding your health care. This is the first one. Do you want your parents here when I ask you some questions about how long ago you first noticed anything…."

Todd realized that if his parents knew he had hidden something from them for months, they would be furious, so he asked them to leave him alone with the doctor. His mother was not pleased; she tried to argue with him but his Dad took her hand and led her out of the room.

"There are going to be a lot of decisions to be made in the next couple of days, Todd", the doctor looked Todd in the eyes. "You don't always have to make them by yourself, and I encourage you to involve your parents as much as possible. This is very hard for them. But perhaps you have something to tell me…."

"Yeah … um … I kinda felt something a couple of months ago. I don't want my parents to know… they'll be really mad … but my Dad was away and my Mom is so stressed … and I was embarrassed, you know…."

The doctor nodded. He knew all too well how difficult it is for kids who are sensitive to what is going on at home.

"Okay, I understand. But for the next little while there are going to be a lot of people looking at your body and asking questions. You are going to be very embarrassed but you'll get used to it. I've got some more questions for you and then your parents need to come back into the room so we can talk about what comes next".

Dr Katz advises:

Testicular cancer, especially for an adolescent, can be very embarrassing and it is not unusual for them to ignore or hide a lump or swelling in that area. There is no screening test for testicular cancer (like mammograms for breast cancer) and there is not good evidence to encourage young men to examine their testicles every month, although advocates for early detection of this cancer support this.

Most testicular cancers are found accidentally, either by the young man himself or a sexual partner. The only established causes for this type of cancer is having an undescended testicle as a toddler or having a family history of testicular cancer. When found early, the success rates for treatments are high; removal of the testicle is almost always necessary and this may be followed by removal of lymph nodes, radiation, or chemotherapy, or some combination of all of these.

What came next was scans and blood tests and a visit with another doctor, Dr Bradbury, who was an urologist. He was tall and a little gruff and he didn't ask Todd if he wanted his parents to be present when he examined him. He had served in Iraq in 2002, he told Todd's father as they shook hands. Todd's mother drew the curtains around the examination table as the doctor asked Todd to lower his pants. She was shocked that the doctor didn't do that but said nothing as she sat back down in the plastic chair.

Thankfully the examination didn't take a lot of time, but Todd's face was bright red as he sat on the edge of the examination table. Dr Bradbury started to talk as he washed his hands at the sink, his back to the family. Vince asked him to repeat what he had said as they couldn't hear him. He used his 'Marine' voice again, and Todd smiled as the doctor turned around and apologized.

"Sorry about that, folks. Well, the good news is that the cancer is localized to the left testicle, and it'll be a simple operation to remove it. The scans suggest that your boy is not going to need any other treatment – no chemo, no radiation. I'd like to get this done as soon as possible. The day after tomorrow sound good to you? My nurse will come in now and get consent for the surgery and tell you some other stuff".

And with that he was gone, the door closing with a bang behind him. Todd felt like he was having an out of body experience. The urologist had not talked directly to him – and he was the one who this was happening to!

Within a few minutes a young woman entered the room. She was wearing blue scrubs and had some papers in her hand.

"Hello everyone! I'm Brit and I work with Dr Bradbury. Don't mind his bedside manner, he's ex-military!"

Vince cleared his throat and his wife elbowed him. He kept quiet but it was not easy.

"My Dad's a Marine!" said Todd.

"Oh gosh, sorry about that", the nurse now looked embarrassed. "Not everyone's used to the 'take no prisoner's approach' but he's a really good surgeon".

Her cheeks were flushed and she took a few seconds to rifle through the papers that she carried.

"Okay, Todd, here's what's going to happen…"

She talked directly to Todd and explained about the surgery and recovery. She explained that the surgeon would place a prosthetic into his scrotum so that no one would be able to tell the difference from what he looked like 'down there' before. Todd's face felt hot and he knew he was as red as a candy apple. He could not look at his parents and so focused on what the nurse was saying, but he still didn't hear all of it. She had some pamphlets for him to read and then she asked if anyone had any questions. Todd's parents shook their heads and Todd, who was still in shock, didn't have any questions either. Both he and his parents signed the consent form and left. Now they just had to wait the two days before the operation.

Dr Katz advises:

Older adolescents have one foot in childhood and the other in young adulthood. They often don't have the maturity to deal with important matters such as their health, but don't want their parents to take over. This can be very stressful for their parents who are still responsible for their well-being and have the life experience to advise them. Providing information to the family requires a delicate balance between respecting the growing autonomy of the adolescent who will receive medical care, and the parent(s) who want control over what is going to happen to their child.

Todd and his parents did not receive the best care in their interaction with the urologist and the nurse. The doctor ignored Todd who is going to be the one having surgery while the nurse ignored his parents in talking about the details of the surgery and recovery. It is not clear if Todd really heard what she explained, and his parents were not involved in the conversation. This can lead to misunderstanding in the future; information should be provided to both the adolescent and parents in a way that they all understand.

The day of the surgery was one that Todd hoped he would forget. He felt sick from fear and his stomach was cramping from not having eaten since midnight. After the surgery he had to stay at the surgical center for a couple of hours. He was in pain and hardly listened to the nurse who gave him the discharge instructions. Luckily his mom was there and she seemed to understand. Within a couple of days he felt much better and when the winter break ended, he was ready to go back to school. He was worried about football practice and having to shower along with the other guys but when he looked at himself in the mirror, he couldn't see anything different. He told no one what had happened, not his coach or his best friend.

He was made captain of the team that semester and he enjoyed the perks that came with that. The other kids at school looked at him as he walked in the hallways. He liked to think that they were talking about him as he passed, but in a good way. He hoped that he would hear about scholarships for college soon; his coach had told him that he had a good chance of getting a 'full ride'.

He was immersed in school and football. He had a lot going on; he had five practices a week and a game on Friday nights. Grade 12 was way harder than the year before, and he was barely coping with his assignments and tests. His Dad had gone back overseas on some sort of special mission and he called at odd hours, so Todd hardly got to speak to him.

Todd missed him a lot, especially now that he was in the final semester of his senior year and was waiting to hear back from the colleges he had applied to.

He hardly thought about the cancer at all. He had been back to see the pediatrician once since the surgery and he was upset that the doctor wanted to have a look at his genitals. He told himself that he would not go back there again, and he didn't. But that did not stop the messages that were left on his phone from the pediatrician. They called him because his Mom was not able to answer her phone when she was in the class-room. He ignored their calls, not picking up when he saw their phone number on the display and deleting the messages they left. They even sent a letter to his home but luckily he found it before his mother got home. He didn't open it and hid it under a pile of t-shirts in his closet. Why did he need to go back to the pediatrician?

Dr Katz advises:

It is important to adhere to the instructions for follow-up visits after being treated for any kind of cancer. Despite the success of treating a low-grade testicular cancer with removal of the testicle without the need for other treatment, recurrence of the cancer is still possible. There are unfortunately no guarantees that the cancer won't come back.

The recommendation is for patients to attend regular follow-up appointments, often with blood tests or imaging studies to monitor whether there are any changes related to a possible return of the can-cer. Any long- or late-side effects can be assessed and suggestions for management of these communicated to the survivor.

Survivors should receive a document that describes what blood tests and/or scans they will need, how often and for how long into the future. This is called a survivorship care plan and it should contain a description of the stage and grade of the cancer, the treatments pro-vided, and details of follow-up monitoring. Information about keeping healthy are also included such as prescriptions for physical activity, maintaining a healthy weight, using sun protection, avoiding alcohol and recreational drugs, coping, etc.

Something that bothered Todd was his relationship with his Mom. Ever since his surgery she kept asking how he was doing. He felt that he was doing fine, but her constant reminding him about the cancer was not helping. She never said it out loud, but she asked how he was in a special way now. Her voice changed and she had this weird look on her face. He was fine, couldn't she see that? He didn't understand why she was so worried. He was playing football, he was coping with schoolwork, and he even kept his room neat. It was now almost four months since his surgery and he wanted to forget it even happened. But she wouldn't let him forget. She had become very attentive to what he was eating. They hardly ate dinner together anymore; he came home late from football practice and she usually ate early because she was famished when she got home just after 4:30 pm. She often left him his dinner on a plate in the fridge, expecting him to warm it in the microwave, but he usually threw it in the garbage. By the time he got home, the salad she had left for him was wilted and looked gross so that went in the garbage too. He mostly ate a bag of microwave popcorn while he did his homework and drank some chocolate milk before he went to bed. Some days he stopped at a drive-through on his way home from practice and had a chicken sandwich and milkshake. His mom could not understand why he was eating fast food and nagged him to eat a decent dinner. She was getting on his nerves, but he didn't say anything to her because he knew that she was worried about him, he just didn't understand why.

His Dad came home a couple of weeks before he graduated high school. They had a lot to celebrate; Todd's team had won the football season, he had received a scholarship to the college of his choice, and he was going to the Prom with Rachel, a classmate he had wanted to date for months but was too busy for a girlfriend. One of the first things his Dad asked about was his health. Todd knew he was going to ask about this and he'd prepared his response.

"I'm really good, Dad. The doc says I don't need to go back to see him anymore! Isn't that great?"

There was something about the way his son answered that just didn't feel right to Vince. He couldn't quite figure out what that was, but he had a feeling that his son was lying to him.

"That sounds good, Todd, but I thought you were going to be followed for 5 years, at least that's what they told your Mom when you had your surgery".

"No, that's not what I remember", said Todd emphatically. He was scrambling to think how he could persuade his father that he did not need to go back for anymore visits.

Todd excused himself and hurried out of the room. Vince decided that he needed to call the pediatrician to find out whether Todd did not need follow-up. As he suspected, the receptionist confirmed that they had not been able to reach Todd. They had called him repeatedly but he never returned their calls. They had even sent a letter but received no response to that either.

When his wife came home after school she looked exhausted. She was teaching Grade 4 and the students were not the most cooperative. They were disrespectful and a lot of her time was spent trying to get through to them. As much as Vince knew she needed some time to decompress, this business with Todd not going for follow-up visits was something they had to talk about.

"Michelle, did you know that Todd has missed visits to the pediatrician?" Vince tried to keep the anger out of his voice.

"What?" his wife looked genuinely shocked.

"I asked Todd how he was doing health-wise and he said he was fine. I asked if he had been back to the doctor and he said he didn't have to..."

"That's nonsense..." Michelle interrupted her husband.

"I thought something was off in his response to me so I called the pediatrician's office and they said that they had called him and also sent a letter but he never called them back. What exactly is going on with that boy?"

Michelle immediately became defensive. She had to take sole responsibility for their son when Vince was away, and she thought that by now Todd should be more mature. Now that he was 18 years old, almost an adult, with a busy schedule she barely saw Todd and she felt guilty that she didn't know about this.

"I thought he knew that he had to see Dr Bateman, his pediatrician! He was right there after the surgery when the nurse talked about the need for follow-up care. He needs some blood tests and also CT scans for 5 years. I thought he knew..."

Her shoulders slumped and she looked defeated.

"It's okay, Michie", Vince called her by her nickname, "We'll have to talk with him and we have to do this together. He needs to know that this is not acceptable. And he can't lie to us either!"

Dr Katz advises:

Two of the milestones that adolescents need to reach during the later teenage years are autonomy and independence. They need to start taking responsibility for their decisions, including about their health. But a diagnosis of cancer is very serious and not following up with health care providers and the necessary monitoring of their disease may result in poor outcomes that can threaten their life. Ignoring phone calls and hiding this from parents is both a breach of trust and dangerous. But it is also a reflection of the adolescent trying to assert power. It may also be a way that the young person tries to move forward and away from the cancer experience. Cancer of this kind carries inherent embarrassment and an adolescent boy may be trying to avoid physical examinations as well as reminders of having cancer.

That afternoon when Todd came home, he found his parents waiting for him at the kitchen table. He no longer had football practice after school and usually went straight to his room after grabbing something from the fridge to eat.

"What's up, parents?" he asked with a smile on his face as he stood in front of the open fridge.

"Todd", Vince's voice was much quieter than usual. This attracted Todd's attention and he immediately turned towards them.

His mother jumped in.

"Todd, why didn't you go for your follow-up appointments?" Her voice was wobbly and she looked like she was going to cry.

"And why did you lie to me when I asked you point blank about this?" Vince was angry and Todd knew he was in big trouble. He was scared when his Dad got angry; it hadn't happened often but it was terrifying to be on the receiving end. He used to feel sorry for any Marine reporting to his Dad who did something wrong.

"I dunno…. I guess I feel okay and I was busy…." His voice grew quieter as he looked at his parents' faces. He could see worry and disappointment in their eyes and now he felt guilty.

His father didn't say anything. Todd could see that he was holding back his words but his mother didn't wait before she yelled at him.

"That is not an excuse, Todd! None of that is! You had CANCER! Think about that for just a minute! It could have KILLED you! It still might!"

They were all shocked at that last bit. Todd thought that after they removed his testicle that he was free and clear; what did she mean when she said that the cancer could still kill him?

"Michie ... Michelle", his father was almost pleading with his wife, "Hang on a minute. Let's talk this through. There's no use yelling and scaring the boy...."

Michelle held her head in her hands. She was crying and her shoulders rocked up and down. She looked at Todd whose face was ashen.

"I'm sorry, honey", she stammered between sobs, "I didn't mean to scare you but I am so scared. I am terrified that if the cancer comes back...." She couldn't say it out loud.

Now it was Todd who could not stop his feelings from erupting.

"I thought that after the surgery I was okay! I don't understand.... What have I done wrong? I just want to have a normal life! I'm sorry if I worried you but I feel fine...."

Todd was crying and his mother got up and out her arms around her son who towered over her by a foot but was still her little boy.

Dr Katz advises:

A diagnosis of cancer is a biographical and social interruption for adolescents and young adults. What was normal life is changed by the illness and some will try to cope by avoiding any mention of the cancer. They may also ignore any interventions necessary to monitor their health when treatment is over. This is not a deliberate intention to hurt those who love them, but rather an attempt to return to what their life was before.

Nothing can prepare a young person for illness at this stage of their life. Thinking that they are invincible and immortal is normal for adolescents, many of whom have never been seriously ill or hurt before. An effective coping mechanism is denial and they may not recall conversations about what needs to happen after treatment. They are not deliberately trying to be oppositional; they are trying to do their best to return to normal. However their parents' approach to after-treatment care may be 180 degrees from this. Parents want to protect their child and want their child to do what their health care team recommends. This often means follow-up visits at frequent intervals in order to catch any signs of recurrence or new side effects as quickly as possible. This can be difficult for an adolescent to understand when all they want is to put the cancer behind them.

Vince looked at his wife and son, hugging each other and crying.

This needs to stop, he thought to himself; he hated it when either of them cried. He took a deep breath.

"Okay, enough of this! We need to talk this out. Stop crying you two!"

Michelle and Todd did just that. They both had small smiles on their face now, very aware of how tears made Vince uncomfortable.

Michelle poured them each a glass of ice water and they sat at the kitchen table, emotions under control, and they talked. Todd admitted that he knew what he was doing was not right; he acknowledged that he felt guilty ignoring the calls from the doctor's orders. Michelle explained to Todd that she was sick with worry that the cancer would come back and that yes, she had not shared that with him before because she thought that he knew that. Vince told them both that he felt guilty that he was away so much and he intended to be more present for them both in the future. He had been considering staying on in the military for a few more years, but this had shown him that he needed to retire from active duty, for all their sakes. It was a good talk and now they had a plan.

Conclusion

Adolescents with cancer face many psychological and social challenges and they attempt to deal with these the best way they know how. This may mean that they ignore instructions about caring for themselves and/ or follow-up care. They may deny what has happened in an attempt to live a 'normal' life. They may also keep their diagnosis a secret from friends out of embarrassment or a desire to not be seen as weak or a victim. This can be frustrating for parents who are aware of what is needed in terms of after-care and surveillance of the cancer. Questioning authority, increasing autonomy, and gaining independence are key tasks of adolescents, and ones that both frighten and challenge parents. Communicating openly, with or without the help of professionals, can help to deal with these challenges.

Reflective Questions

After reading this story:

- How can denying the cancer, a common response in adolescents, have negative effects on the young person and their family?
- How could Todd's mother have handled the situation better?
- What could the doctor's office have done about Todd's ignoring their messages beyond repeated phone calls and sending a letter?
- What could Todd's father Vince have done differently in this situation?

7

THE UNSPEAKABLE

"IT'S TOO SOON FOR HIM TO LEAVE US"

Neil and Jared have been a couple since their college days. They are now both 32 years old and were married on a beach in Mexico two years ago. Neil is an artist who uses mixed media to create streetscapes that have sold well at galleries and art shows. Jared, his husband, is a registered nurse who works in a pediatric unit at a large hospital near where they live. Neil came out to his parents in high school; his mother Lisa always suspected that her son was gay and was thankful when he eventually told them and there were no longer any secrets in the family. Dave, Neil's father, was less happy but over the years has come to terms with his son's sexuality; he liked Jared from the moment they met. Neil has an older sister, Amanda, who recently got engaged to her partner Lance. Amanda and Neil have always been close and she has known he was gay since he was in his early teens. Amanda and Neil live on opposite coasts but they talk often and the two couples have vacationed together.

One year ago, Neil started having headaches that were so bad he had to stop working in his studio. He didn't tell Jared who would have panicked and made him go to the Emergency Department. But then he fell a

DOI: 10.4324/9781003242680-7

couples of times, once when alone in their condo and another time when they went for a walk. Jared was worried but Neil assured him it was because he was wearing new sneakers. When Neil started to forget the simplest things, like where he had put the keys to his studio or when his next exhibition was to take place, Jared talked to one of the doctors at the hospital who encouraged him to insist that Neil see a doctor. Neil agreed reluctantly, and after a whirlwind of tests they met with a neurologist.

The diagnosis was awful; Neil had a glioblastoma multiforme, an aggressive brain cancer, that is almost always lethal. Neil's family was devastated. Amanda postponed her wedding indefinitely. Jared was going to take a leave from work but his mother-in-law persuaded him to hold off for the time being. Lisa had retired soon after Neil and Jared were married and she wanted to take care of Neil, even though initially he was doing quite well. Neil had surgery to remove the tumor in his brain, but as the doctors anticipated, they were not able to get all of it out. Radiation followed that shrunk what was left of the tumor and he started chemotherapy. They were told that the chemotherapy would not cure the cancer but would slow progression.

Dr Katz advises:

Glioblastoma multiforme is an aggressive cancer that can be managed but there is no cure for this cancer. Most people diagnosed with this cancer unfortunately succumb to it within a year of diagnosis, despite treatment. The tumor tends to spread throughout the brain and symptoms develop based on where this spread goes.

Symptoms associated with this cancer include headaches, nausea or vomiting, confusion, difficulties with speech and balance, blurred vision and other visual problems, loss of bladder control, and seizures. Irritability and personality changes are also possible and may impact relationships and social support.

Nine months later Neil started to develop new symptoms and scans confirmed that the cancer was growing. There were times when he was confused and didn't recognize some of their friends who had offered to stay with Neil so that Jared could get some respite. Shortly after, Jared took a leave from his position at the hospital. His supervisor was supportive and told him that he was a valued member of the team and that he would always have a place in the unit. She was almost in tears when she talked to him and Jared left before he started to cry. This time when Neil's mother suggested she could take care of Neil, Jared told her with some irritation in his voice, that he and Neil were partners, in sickness and in health, and he would be the primary caregiver for her son. This was just the beginning of tension between Jared and his in-laws.

Neil continued to decline and it was hard for everyone to watch. He went to see the oncologist every two weeks. It was getting increasingly difficult to get him out of bed, into a wheelchair and then into the car. Jared was strong but Neil was tall and now he didn't have the strength to help lift himself. Making things even worse was that Neil was now quick to anger, and he often shouted at Jared when his partner tried to help him. Often his words did not make sense and Jared struggled to understand him. Neil seemed unaware of how weak he was and how difficult it was to move him into the car. Jared used every bit of patience to deal with these outbursts but he didn't share this with Neil's family. It seemed like a betrayal; they had this image of Neil as a kind person, as he was in the 'before' times. Jared wasn't sure that Lisa and Dave would even believe him and he was scared that they would somehow make him the bad guy in the situation. He kept quiet and tried to manage on his own.

Neil's parents came with the couple to his next appointment with the oncologist. They were shocked by how much worse he was and wanted to talk to the doctor. Jared was dreading this; at previous appointments, Lisa had gone into 'Mom' mode and asked too many questions. And Dave had just sat there, appearing at times to be in another world. This appointment was not any different and in fact, was worse than Jared expected.

Lisa started the appointment by telling the oncologist and the nurse practitioner who worked with him that she had a list of questions that she wanted answered.

"I want to know EVERYTHING about what is happening with my son!"

Jared cringed; he had told his in-laws everything that he knew and she was suggesting that he had kept information from them. Neil was sitting in a wheelchair next to Jared. He didn't seem to be listening to what was going on and hadn't reacted to his mother's outburst.

"Honey…" Dave tried to calm his wife down, but there was no stopping her.

"Firstly, why did you stop the chemotherapy? He was perfectly fine until you stopped that! How did that happen? Who agreed to that?"

Her voice was shrill and Jared could only sit there, his face growing more and more red, his hands clenched.

"I was doing some research and Neil has not had all the treatments available! Why is he not having that electric field treatment? And there are those things that you put into his brain that deliver chemo to the tumor! Why can't you do that?"

Lisa sank back into the chair. Her mouth was dry and her heart was beating very fast. She was a little short of breath as searched in her purse for a bottle of water.

The oncologist, Dr Lane, paused as if gathering her thoughts. She was a small woman in her early forties, with large tortoise shell glasses that covered her brown eyes. She had a reputation in the hospital of being 'small but mighty', a fierce advocate for her patients and her team. Jared really liked her and trusted that she was doing the best she could with Neil and his awful cancer. She always returned Jared's calls and was patient in explaining to him what was happening about Neil's response to treatment.

"Mrs Markham, Mr Markham, Jared and Neil…" She looked at each of them as she spoke their name. "I hear your concern and I understand how difficult this is for all of you. I'm going to start at the beginning of Neil's treatment…"

When he heard the doctor say his name, Neil looked at her and then at Jared. He seemed confused to have heard his name and he had a questioning facial expression. Jared leaned over and whispered in his ear, "We're at the doctor's office, don't be scared, nothing bad is going to happen."

Jared held Neil's hand, his tanned fingers holding tight to Neil's long, artist's fingers, now almost translucent with prominent blue veins running along the bones.

Dr Lane described the findings of the scans, the surgery performed by her colleague, and the radiation therapy. The medical team knew that this was not a cure, but rather a way to buy more time. Then there was the chemotherapy that held off further changes, but only for a while. And now here they were. Neil was not going to get better and there was no hope of a cure, not even with experimental treatments.

"There has to be more that you can do!!!! Please try something... more surgery, more radiation, more chemo, different chemo.... It's too soon for him to leave us!"

Neil was looking at his mother who was crying. His father had his hand on her arm as if holding her back from doing something. Jared was holding tight to Neil's hand and his hand was shaking.

"Lisa, no!" Jared's voice was louder than he intended but he was horrified at what she was demanding of Dr Lane. "We discussed this with Neil after the chemotherapy and he said that he was okay with stopping the chemo when it wasn't working. Don't you remember?"

"Honey, you must remember! We were sitting in Neil's bedroom and he told us..." Dave tried to reason with his wife. Part of him knew it was useless to try and persuade her, but he agreed with Jared. Neil had told them all that he didn't want more treatment if it was futile.

A flash of irritation went through Jared's mind. Neil's bedroom? It was THEIR bedroom but it now seemed like he didn't count, as least not for Lisa. As a pediatric nurse he knew how protective mothers could be, but he and Neil were a couple, and his role should not be diminished or ignored.

The nurse practitioner, Adam, took the brief pause to ask a question.

"Folks, there's an advance directive in Neil's chart. I believe Neil signed this when he first came to the hospital for the surgery. That might clear up some of the issues about more treatment. Can we take a moment to review that?"

Dr Lane breathed out; this was more difficult than she anticipated.

Adam pulled up the document that had been scanned into Neil's chart. Neil had signed the directive giving Jared the authority to make medical decisions for him when he was no longer able to. He knew that in the future he might not be able to make decisions and he wanted Jared as his husband to take over. He and Jared had talked about what he wanted for medical care and life-extending interventions; he wanted this in writing so that his wishes would be carried out if and when the time came.

Dr Katz advises:

Advance care planning, or having an advance directive, allows a person to state what they want at or near the end of life when they cannot speak for them self or are unable to make decisions about their care. This is a legal document that goes into effect only if someone cannot speak for them self. It is a 'living' document that the individual can make changes to as the situation changes over time. This document gives direction to medical providers about things like tube feeding, being resuscitated, and/or being put on a ventilator.

There are additional documents that can be completed in addition to the advance directive. These include a living will that tells medical care providers how the person wants to be treated depending on specific circumstances if they are unconscious and cannot make decisions. A durable power of attorney for health care is a legal document that names a health care proxy, someone who makes medical decisions if the person cannot. The health care proxy should be someone who knows the values of the person and there should be a sharing of these values and the decisions that this proxy can make if an advance care directive has not been created.

Additional information about this can be found from the National Institute on Aging, a division of the US Department of Health and Human Services (https://www.nia.nih.gov/health/advance-care-planning-health-care-directives).

Neil's parents were surprised that Neil had an advance directive; they did not know about this.

"So, let me understand this," began Dave. His voice was shaky and he hesitated before continuing. "Neil, our son, has given YOU the power to make decisions about his care?"

He looked at Jared with an angry expression on his face. His feelings about Neil coming out years ago resurfaced and Jared was the target for his anger at what had happened to his son even though he liked Jared.

Jared remained silent. He did not want to inflame the situation, but he was angry at Neil for not telling his parents what was in his advance directive when he signed it months ago.

Dr Lane tried to calm things down. "Let's all take a deep breath here, please! I understand that this is difficult, but your son signed a legal document and we have to abide by his wishes. Let's focus on how best to meet Nail's needs now and in the future."

Jared spoke, his voice soft and almost pleading.

"Dave, Lisa. Please let's stop this! Neil signed the advance directive because he knew how hard it would be for you to make difficult decisions because you love him! Neil knew that despite how hard this would be, I have the medical background to understand things related to his condition. I don't want to fight about this. I want to respect Neil's wishes no matter how much it hurts."

Neil was looking at Jared and then at his parents and back again. The deterioration in his speech was frustrating for him, as well as for his family, but Jared could interpret his facial expressions.

"Neil, baby, do you understand what we've been talking about?" Jared's voice was almost a whisper.

Neil nodded and a tear rolled down his cheek. Jared wiped the tear away and took his hand again. Despite their anger and frustration Lisa and Dave knew that Jared loved their son very much and that it was reciprocated.

"Adam, I'm going to leave you to talk about supports and resources," Dr Lane was heading to the door. "I am always available if you have questions or a new symptom to report. I have to leave you now to start my clinic but Adam can give you all sorts of information. I will continue to see Neil every two weeks, unless something happens that needs my attention."

As the door closed Adam moved his chair to sit closer to Neil. He talked directly to him and Neil's eyes stared at him with more focus than Jared had seen in weeks.

"Okay, Neil. I know that this appointment has been hard, not just for you, but for everyone. Your family loves you a lot, but you know that, right?"

Neil nodded and whispered "Yes".

"We need to talk about what you want as things get worse. I know this is hard to talk about but this is happening to you and you get to decide what you want and where you want to be. So I'm going to ask a bunch of questions and you can nod or shake your head. Is that okay?"

Neil nodded again and Jared squeezed his hand.

Adam asked a lot of questions and Neil was able to say a few words in response. The plan was for him to stay at home, with Jared providing most of his care. His parents would visit as often as they wanted, but they had to call first. If Jared needed help, they would be the first ones he contacted. Jared agreed that when it felt right, he would also welcome assistance from the hospice program.

Lisa and Dave did not say much but as Adam talked. They looked at each other as he asked questions and laid out the plan. They were not happy with all control going to Jared. But Neil seemed to agree and they had to live with his decisions. At least for the time being...

Dr Katz advises:

Tension or outright conflict can arise when parents of a young adult have to share care with the partner of the person with cancer. An advance directive can be helpful to lay out the wishes of the person with cancer, but legality does not take away hurt feelings and different opinions. The goal should be to support each other and work toward meeting the needs of the person who needs care.

This is a distressing situation for all concerned, and tempers will flare and the parents or partner may choose to 'pull rank" in order to influence the other. This is futile and will ultimately be detrimental to everyone, especially the person who is vulnerable and needs support and care.

An objective professional such as a social worker, nurse, or case manager may be able to put the needs of the person first and communicate this to the family. Reminding them to put their own feelings second to the task at hand – caring for their loved one who is close or at the end of life – can help to avoid arguments or manage conflict better.

For the next two months, Jared and Neil's parents worked together to care for him. First Jared slept next to Neil in their bed but when he started to have convulsions quite regularly despite medication, he ordered a hospital bed to be set up in the living room. Lisa started to sleep over on the couch and Jared was grateful to be able to get a few hours of uninterrupted sleep. When Lisa went home in the morning to shower and get some rest, Jared bathed his partner and sorted out his medications for the day. Amanda, Neil's sister, traveled from the East Coast to visit. She stayed a few days and wasn't much help. She was shocked by Neil's condition and told Jared that she couldn't bear to see him like this. She was taking the easy way out and was going home. Jared hugged her, told her he understood, and said he supported her decision.

As the days passed, Neil seemed to go into another world. In the beginning he slept most of the time, helped by the pain medication Dr Lane had ordered. Lisa and Dave had moved in and the three of them took turns staying close by his bedside. It was not easy; Jared felt that both Lisa and Dave resented his ability to give Neil his medications, including injections that they could not. Jared also continued to bathe Neil every day, and Dave thought this was unnecessary and also a bit weird. When he mentioned this to Lisa, she told him in no uncertain terms that it was HE who was weird for thinking that. Spoken and unspoken feelings swirled around.

In the last few days of his life, Neil became more agitated and had lost any ability to respond to questions or instructions. He thrashed around in the bed and nothing any of them did could calm him. Jared had seen people in this stage and called in the hospice team despite some resistance from Neil's parents. They offered medication to calm him and that helped; Jared and his in-laws kept a constant vigil, someone always holding his hand. Jared took the midnight shift and nodded off around 2 am in the morning. When something woke him suddenly, he realized that Neil's hand was cold. He put his head on Neil's chest, over his heart, and it was still.

Dr Katz advises:

In the last days at the end of life, people are often non-responsive and may exhibit behaviors that look like they are in pain and suffering. This is called terminal agitation and is a sign that death is near. It is often more distressing for those who are watching what is happening than it is for the person at the end of life. Medication can be given to calm the person and make them more comfortable, but these medications are also sedating.

Some family members may question if these medications are addictive because they are the kind of medications that are often abused. This is absolutely not the case in this type of situation and to withhold these medications will make things worse for those caring for the person as well as to the one who is in the process of dying.

Jared spent a few minutes with Neil before waking Lisa and Dave. An older nurse had once told him that in some countries when a death has occurred, a window should be opened to allow the person's soul to leave. Jared was not a religious person but he opened the window and the room filled with the cool night air. He walked slowly to the bedroom that he and Neil had shared to wake Neil's parents.

The next weeks were awful. There was the funeral to plan and Jared left it to Neil's parents to organize. It was nothing like Neil had wanted but Jared was too exhausted to fight with them. Amanda tried to comfort Jared as best as she could, but he was grieving so deeply that she couldn't reach him. He went through the motions for the next month, mostly sitting on their bed that he could not bring himself to sleep in. Amanda had organized for the hospital bed to be returned and Jared lay on the couch most nights, eyes wide open in the dark, replaying the memories of his life with Neil. He hardly saw Lisa and Dave, and after Amanda left, all contact with them ended.

Six weeks after Neil died, Jared went back to work. The days were long and lonely and he felt himself getting more and more depressed. He was welcomed back to the unit where he had worked before and within a week or two was back up to speed. The work was a distraction for him, and he found himself immersed in the routines of caring for children who needed full time support.

Dr Katz advises:

There is no timetable on grief and everyone will mourn in their own way, taking their own time. To mourn alone is even more difficult and it is common for depression to follow. The company of family and friends can bring comfort and most religions and cultures have rituals for mourning designed to help those who are left behind.

When there is conflict between members of the family, grief and loss can compound and further complicate feelings. Some people will judge others who they feel are not sad enough or are disrespectful of their adapting to the loss of a loved one. The rifts caused by these actions may be long lasting and yet another loss in the lives of all concerned.

Seeking help to address these issues, whether from a religious leader, a counselor or therapist, or trusted friends can help individuals to accept that everyone is different in their coping and there is no right or wrong way to mourn.

The days and weeks flew by and in a flash, six months had gone by. One day in the cafeteria he sat down at an empty table and was interrupted by one of the resident doctors.

"Is this seat taken?" a deep voice asked, "Is that not the cheesiest pickup line ever?"

Jared looked up as the man sat down opposite him. Pickup line? What was this?

Within minutes they were deep in conversation, and to his surprise, Jared found himself agreeing to have a drink with him later that evening. One drink led to dinner and then a picnic in the park. Soon they were seeing each other whenever their schedules allowed. About a month later, Jared told Amanda that he was seeing someone. She was a little surprised as it was only seven months since Neil had died but from her semi-regular calls with him, she knew how lonely he was. She must have told her parents because shortly after that, Lisa and Dave asked to meet with him. He was dreading this but had no idea what they wanted to talk about. He suggested that they talk on the phone but they insisted on meeting him at the condo.

Things did not go well. Dave was angry with Jared but it was not clear exactly why he felt this way. Lisa cried from the moment they walked into the condo. Jared was not sure what they wanted but as they walked around, Lisa pointed at pieces of art that Neil had created and Dave started piling them up next to the door. Jared was speechless for the first few minutes but then he exploded.

"What are you doing? Stop that! That does NOT belong to you! Did you not hear me? Put that down. NOW!!"

Dave ignored him and continued to remove painting and drawings from the walls in the living room and then Jared's bedroom. Jared followed him.

"Get OUT of my room! You have no right! Get out! Get out!"

Dave ignored him.

Lisa was going through the large bookcase in the study. She was pulling books haphazardly off the shelves and some of them were falling onto the floor.

"Lisa! STOP!" Jared was screaming now. His face was red and he felt as if he were going insane. What were they doing? He reached for his phone and pressed the number for Amanda in his contacts. She answered before he knew what he was going to say.

"Amanda! You have to talk to them! They're tearing up the condo. They're taking everything! All of Neil's stuff! Please! PLEASE!"

"What are you talking about, Jared?" Amanda was shouting into the phone. "Who is 'they'? Are you being robbed?"

"It's your PARENTS!!!!! They're pulling stuff off the walls and the bookcases! All of Neil's paintings! And the books I gave him! All of it! Help me!"

He was crying now and saliva was running down his chin.

"Let me talk to them, Jared! Put my mom on the phone."

Jared handed Lisa the phone. She continued to pull books off the shelves as she talked to her daughter.

"Amanda, now you listen to me! This.... This belongs to Neil! I don't care what the damn will says! This is all we have left of him and his so-called husband is not going to stop us! And what a husband he is too! Already moving on... new boyfriend! So much for his great love!"

Jared could hear Amanda trying to reason with her mother. He could make out the words 'lawyer' and 'trouble' and finally 'police'. Dave had come into the room. In his arms were many of Neil's clothes, the t-shirts splattered with paint and the ripped jeans that Neil loved so much. Jared had not been able to get rid of them and his heart contracted when he saw how carelessly Dave was carrying them. He lunged at his father-in-law and tried to pull them out of his arms. The clothes flew into the air and landed on the furniture and the floor. Jared tried to gather them up, finally crawling between the chairs and the couch to find them all.

Jared could hear Amanda yelling at her mother.

"Mom. Stop it! You can't do this! Neil left his art to Jared! You have plenty of his work! This is not fair! What you are doing is not right! Where's Dad?"

Lisa looked at her husband who was standing across the room.

"Give me the phone, Lisa! Amanda?"

He put the phone on speaker and they listened as Amanda tried to talk sense into them.

"Dad, Mom", she began. Her voice was measured and firm.

"You both know the instructions in Neil's will. He left all his art to Jared. There is no negotiation about that. The condo belongs to Jared and you have to leave now."

Lisa tried to say something but Jared grabbed the phone from Dave's hand. He held it up as Amanda continued.

"What you are doing is not right. You cannot take anything that is not yours. I know it's hard and I wish I was there.... You have to leave now. Neil would not want you to do this to Jared. Listen to me. This is not what Neil would want."

Somehow Amanda's words got through to the couple. Lisa was now crying and Dave looked embarrassed. Jared's heart was beating so fast he could feel his chest shuddering. Dave looked around the room then looked at Jared and shook his head. He put his hand on Lisa's elbow and walked out of the condo, leaving the door open behind them.

Amanda's voice reached Jared's ears.

"I'm so sorry, Jared," her voice sounded so far away, "I'm really sorry. They're just grieving..."

I am too, he thought as he disconnected the call, I am too.

Conclusion

The mere thought of one's child having a cancer that will one day kill them, no matter how old or young the child, is the worst thing that parents could imagine. It is more complicated when the child is older and has a partner; rivalries may occur at the worst possible times. There should be no competition about who loves the person with cancer more, who is better able to provide care, or whose grief is the most valid or real. In the aftermath, everyone suffers and this should draw loved ones closer, not push them apart.

Reflective Questions

After reading this story:

- Both the nurse practitioner and the oncologist were witness to strains in the relationship between the patient's parents and his partner. How could they have intervened in the situation?
- What could Jared have done in the situation when Neil's parents tried to ignore his wishes?
- What could bring this family together after all that has happened?
- What advice would you offer to a family you know who was in a similar situation?

8

KEY TASKS FOR ADOLESCENTS

"I'M NOT A BABY! WHY CAN'T THEY LET ME BE ME"?

Jackie's family was shaken when, a year ago when she was just 15 years old, she was diagnosed with an ovarian germ cell tumor. Deb, her mother, is a registered nurse who works part-time at doctor's office. She had never heard of this type of tumor and thought that ovarian cancer only happens to women in later life. Jackie's symptoms were also strange; her abdomen was swollen but she did not seem to be gaining weight in other places of her body. The school nurse at Jackie's high school noticed this and her first thought was that Jackie was pregnant. Jackie was horrified and started crying when the nurse questioned her; she was upset about this change in her body and had started to wear baggy tops to hide her shape. The school nurse called Jackie's parents who took her to see their primary care provider. Dr Brandon was mystified and sent Jackie to the lab for some blood tests. The physical exam she did suggested something on one of Jackie's ovaries. She made a referral to a specialist at a nearby cancer center.

The specialist, a gynecologic-oncologist named Dr Shah, ordered a series of tests, including ones that could suggest the presence of ovarian

DOI: 10.4324/9781003242680-8

cancer. She also ordered a CT scan and MRI to determine the extent of the cancer and whether it had spread. The tests confirmed the presence of cancer in her left ovary. Fortunately the tumor was small and had not spread. Jackie had laparoscopic surgery to remove the ovary as well as the uterine tube; her uterus and the other ovary and uterine tube were healthy and did not need to be removed. The pathology found it was a germ cell tumor. Jackie recovered physically but everything had happened so fast that she barely understood exactly what she had gone through. She went back to school two weeks after the surgery and acted as if nothing had happened.

Dr Katz advises:

Ovarian germ cell tumors occur in teenage girls and most often affect only one of the ovaries. This cancer is not easy to diagnose because there are usually no symptoms in the early stages. One symptom, swelling of the abdomen without weight gain, should be regarded with suspicion. Investigations include a CT and/or MRI scan and a surgical procedure (laparotomy) to confirm the cancer; samples of tissue are usually taken to be examined by a pathologist. Blood tests are also helpful to look for certain tumor markers; alpha fetoprotein or human chorionic gonadotrophin (HCG) levels may be raised, indicating the presence of ovarian cancer.

Treatment is provided based on the stage and grade of the cancer. Surgery is usually performed and involves removal of the ovary where the cancer is found as well as the uterine tube on one or both sides. The uterus may also be removed and for some women, radiation and chemotherapy may also be needed. The latter treatments usually result in the women being unable to have children in the future.

After the surgery Jackie seemed more moody but her parents thought this was part of her being a teenager. She had always been quiet and didn't often invite friends to come over. Her father Mike owned a fast food franchise and he worked long hours. He was usually not home for dinner and they rarely ate together as a family. Jackie's younger sister Andrea was 12 and the athletic one in the family; their mother almost always went to watch her practices and games and so dinner for Jackie was usually eaten in her room while she did her homework. Jackie also spent a lot of time online; she played video games with people from all over the world and they were her friends, rather than the kids at school.

One evening her mother came home early from Andrea's basketball practice. Jackie heard the backdoor slam and her mother's loud footsteps as she climbed the stairs.

"Jackie! Jacqueline Masters!"

When her mother called her by her full name it always meant she was in trouble.

"Open this door right now, Miss!"

Jackie removed her headphones and paused the game she was playing. She opened her bedroom door and her mother almost fell into the room.

"What's up, Mom?" Jackie stood with her back to her desk, her arms crossed.

"You sit down young lady!" Her mother had her 'nurse' voice on full volume.

"I got a call from your home room teacher while I was at Andy's practice…. He said you have been missing class and you were caught smoking behind the gym!"

Jackie scrambled to think of what to say. She knew that when her Mom got worked up about something, it was better to not say much.

"Um, what exactly did Mr Pooper say?"

"Mr PORTER", her mother emphasized the teacher's proper name, "Mr Porter told me exactly that. You have been missing class and you were caught smoking! Just exactly what do you think you are doing?"

Jackie shrugged and looked at the monitor where trolls and monsters moved back and forth.

"Just wait till your father gets home!" fumed Deb as she left the room. They had never had any kind of trouble from Jackie before. Why was this happening?

When Mike got home it was close to 10 pm. Deb was too tired to get into the whole story and decided to leave it till the morning. But he was gone by 7 am and she still had not talked to him. She sat at the kitchen table for a long time after the girls had left for school. She reached for her phone and called Jackie's high school, hoping that Mr Porter would be available to talk to her.

"Mrs Masters, good morning!" The teacher sounded very cheerful for someone who had to face 30 or more teenagers every day.

"I'm sorry to bother you, Mr Porter, but I have some additional questions about Jackie…. I was so shocked yesterday that I wasn't thinking…."

"I expected a call from you", the teacher replied, "Our call yesterday…"
Deb interrupted him.

"Yes, the call. You have to understand that we have never had a moment's trouble from Jackie and now this. It's so strange and of course very upsetting to us…."

There was a pause before the teacher responded.

"I understand … the change in Jackie has not gone unnoticed by staff here recently. Has anything changed at home?"

Now it was Deb's turn to hesitate. Jackie did not want anyone to know about her surgery and so her parents had not told anyone outside of their immediate family. Both Deb and Mike had tried to persuade Jackie to at least let the school know, but she was insistent that her parents not say anything to anyone. But something had changed in Jackie and Deb needed to get to the bottom of this out of the ordinary behavior. Missing school was bad enough, but smoking? She had to tell Mr Porter the truth.

"Um, Mr Porter, Jackie had some surgery a while back … you remember she was off school for two weeks? Well, she seemed fine and that's why what you said yesterday is so shocking to us. The surgery was three months ago…"

"Hmmm…." The teacher thought for a moment. He recalled that she had missed those two weeks, but she came back to class and had acted normally. He had checked with a few of Jackie's teachers and they said that it was just in the last three or four weeks that she had started missing class. And then a few days before he had smelled smoke when he checked that the gym doors were locked. When he looked out the door he saw Jackie and two other girls talking to some of the senior boys; they all rushed off when they saw him. He found a smoldering cigarette butt in the grass where they had been gathered.

"Mrs Masters, I think the problem stems from the kids Jackie has started hanging round with … um…. Well, kids that perhaps are not a good influence".

Deb put her head in hands as he continued to talk. She had always feared that Jackie was a follower rather than a leader and that trouble would result. And here they were, with Jackie in trouble. What would come next?

Dr Katz advises:

Adolescence is a time when friends become the most important influence in life, taking over from parents and other family members. Teenagers need to feel that they belong to a social group and this becomes the focus of their life. Common interests, such as playing video games, serve to cement social bonds and the teenager begins to look outside the family for validation and support.

Behaviors that are out of the ordinary for a teenage child are common and the result of social influences that often do not concur with the values of the family. The teenager tests the boundaries of what they can and cannot do, and what they can get away with. This is both exciting and terrifying for the young person who may feel guilty about what they are doing, while at the same time almost enjoying their parents' disapproval and distress.

This is a difficult time for parents who may fear that their child will get into worse trouble or pull away from them altogether. And often parents forget that they too went through this, perhaps with less danger or outward defiance.

Deb called her husband and told him that they needed to talk about Jackie and he promised to get home earlier than usual. They sat outside on the deck where neither of their girls could overhear their conversation. Mike was shocked that his oldest daughter could have done what his wife told him.

"But she's always been so good, such a great example for Andrea..." he protested.

"Well, she's certainly NOT a great example right now!" replied his wife, anger in her voice. Mike could never hear anything critical about Jackie; she was his golden girl.

"We have to do something about this, Mike! I tried talking to her and was met with a stare and then she just ignored me! You need to talk to her! Maybe you can get through to her that this is NOT okay!"

Mike nodded, got up and went into the house. The thoughts in his head whirled around; what was he going to say to her?

He knocked on her door and waited what seemed to be an overly long time before she called out for him to enter. While he waited, he heard the sounds of drawers opening and closing and the whispers of bedsheets being moved.

"Honey? Jackie?" He looked at his daughter who was sitting on her bed, her eyes glaring at him. He had never seen her like this! Where was his golden girl?

Mike did not get much further with her than his wife had the previous day. She was belligerent and rude and for a moment he felt like shaking her. He had never touched any of the women in his family in anger before and he was not going to start now. He left her room with a sick feeling in his stomach. How was he going to tell Deb that he had failed?

The next evening while Andrea was at practice, Deb decided that she was going to have it out with Jackie. Mike was such a pushover when it came to Jackie that he was no help at all so Deb was going to address this herself. Once again she was met with silence when she tried to talk to Jackie. She warned her that there would be severe consequences if she did not go to school and the smoking had to stop.

"Do you understand what I just said?" Deb demanded of her daughter.

"Yeeesssss, Mom!" was the response.

"I mean it, Jackie! And don't try and get around your Dad by playing the 'poor little me' card. He is one hundred percent in agreement with me. This behavior has to change!"

With a sigh, Deb walked away, shaking her head. Jackie was used to getting her own way with Mike. The few times they had to discipline her over the years, Jackie had tried to get her Dad to change his mind or see things her way. But this was not going to happen this time; Deb was determined to put a stop to this.

The following weeks seemed to go more smoothly. Deb checked in with Mr Porter and he reported that Jackie had not missed class. What he didn't tell her was that she had changed the way she was dressing. He wasn't sure that her mother didn't know this and he didn't want to appear to be noticing her appearance; that might be misconstrued. But Jackie certainly looked different these days. She was wearing ripped black jeans and a long black coat, even when it was hot outside. Her eyes were rimmed in dark black and she had started wearing black lipstick along with copious amounts of white face powder. She looked nothing like the shy girl she used to be.

One evening Mike suggested that he and Deb go for a walk after dinner. He had once again come home early from work and Deb had a feeling that there was something related to Jackie that he wanted to talk about.

"Deb, I don't want you to think that I'm crazy but I think I saw Jackie today, and she looked like a stranger…." He was having difficulty getting the words out.

"What do you mean, Mike? She's been so much better! Mr Porter said that she hasn't missed class again…."

Mike cleared his throat.

"I saw her, at least I think it was her, and she was dressed all in black with horrible makeup … she looked like one of those kids… what are they called? Goth. That's it! She looked like she was one of those Goth weirdoes!"

Deb had seen Jackie and Andrea leave for school that morning. She was sure that Jackie was wearing blue jeans and a pink hoodie. And makeup? Deb had not seen a trace of anything on her daughter's face when she left. Maybe her husband was mistaken? She sure hoped he was!

Things got worse that afternoon. The oncologist's office called and said that Jackie had missed an appointment the day before. What appointment, Deb wondered. She didn't have anything marked in her calendar until the next week. What was going on?

"Let's go talk to her! Right now, Mike!"

As Deb anticipated, Jackie denied everything. She told her Dad he was mistaken when he told her he had seen her walking past his shop. She acted offended when her mother suggested that she changed her clothes after she left the house in the morning. And she told them that if Andrea had told them anything, she was a liar and would pay for ratting her out.

"One more thing", Deb looked like she was going to cry. "Did you change your appointment with Dr Shah?"

"What appointment?" was Jackie's reply.

"Don't lie to us, Jackie! This is serious! This is your health we're talking about!" Deb had reached the end of her rope. She could tell that Jackie was lying and this hurt more than the denial about her appearance.

Dr Katz advises:

Adolescents should begin to learn to be self-sufficient and to make decisions for themselves, but this doesn't mean that they will make good decisions or behave responsibly. Some will be defiant and oppositional and put themselves at risk, physically or emotionally. It can be difficult for them to admit to doing things that are dangerous or merely stupid. Confronting them with facts can lead to more lies in order to preserve their sense of independence.

Socializing with new friends who their parents may think are unsuitable is a form of pushing boundaries, another way that they try to assert their independence. In order to fit in, teenagers will often change their appearance, with clothing choices an easy way to do this. Tattoos and facial piercings may follow, so perhaps makeup and clothing are the least problematic!

Ignoring things that remind them of any kind of weakness or vulnerability is another way that teens attempt to assert their autonomy. Missing medical appointments is one way of doing this; teenagers who are diabetic often neglect their self-monitoring with severe consequences. This is all part of growing up, but parents are justified in being worried about this.

Mike managed to negotiate a truce between the three of them. Deb rescheduled the appointment with the oncologist and Jackie attended with her mother, even though she was sulky and almost rude to the doctor. Everything was fine – the blood tests for tumor markers were normal and there was no sign of the cancer on physical examination. Dr Shah tried to engage Jackie in conversation but received only nods or grunts in response. Deb had to bite her tongue on the drive home; she wanted to yell at her daughter about how rude she had been, but she knew that this would only cause more problems.

But the truce did not last long. One weekend morning while Jackie was still asleep, Andrea came into the kitchen where Mike and Deb were having coffee. Now Andrea was acting strangely.

"Please not her too! I don't think I can take it if Andrea also starts acting strangely!" Deb thought to herself.

Andrea had something to say but she could barely get the words out.

"Mom, Dad, I shouldn't be telling you this, but I'm scared...." She looked terrified.

"What is it, honey? What's wrong? Has something happened? You can tell us anything. We won't get mad, I promise you!" Now Deb looked scared.

"Let the child talk, Deb!" Mike was also worried; what would their youngest say?

"Okay, so it's about Jackie and she'll kill me if she knew I was telling you this ... she has a boyfriend! He's 21 and he's kinda weird..."

Deb and Mike looked at each other. A boyfriend was one thing, but he was four years older than her! They thanked Andrea for telling them and promised that they would not tell Jackie where they had heard about this. They needed to figure out how they were going to deal with this newest issue.

The opportunity presented itself in a way that neither of them anticipated. Mike came home one afternoon while Deb was at work; there was a vehicle parked in the driveway that he did not recognize. It was a large truck with what looked like a condom hanging from the rearview mirror. Mike shook his head in disgust as he opened the front door very quietly. He walked down the hallway toward Jackie's bedroom and stopped a few paces away from the door. The distinctive smell of marijuana was overwhelming.

He knocked on the door and tried to open it at the same time; the door was locked. He heard voices from inside the room, panicked voices and lots of 'shushing'. He knocked again, this time shouting to Jackie to open the door.

She did so a few moments later; the smell of marijuana was intense even with the windows wide open. He looked at his daughter, his golden girl, who at least had the honesty to look guilty as she stood against the open window. The sound of the truck starting was all the proof he needed.

"Jackie!" He sounded more hurt than angry and this made his daughter's eyes fill with tears that she brushed away with the back of her hands.

"Dad ...." Jackie sounded scared.

"I can't talk right now, Jackie", Mike's voice was sad, "Your mother and I will speak to you later".

Deb was furious when she heard what had happened. Her immediate impulse was to confront Jackie, but Mike urged her to wait until they had a plan. They needed to figure out how they were going to talk to her and what they would do if she once again refused to talk to them. Mike had been thinking about what to say all afternoon but he was not sure that anything he said would come out right.

Jackie looked at her parents as they entered her bedroom. She was sitting on the bed and there was no smell of marijuana, replaced instead by the sweet smell of a candle burning on her desk.

"Mom, Dad …." she started to talk but Mike stopped her.

"Jackie, your mother and I are going to do the talking and you are going to do the listening. And when we are done, you are going to do exactly what we tell you. Do you understand?"

Jackie nodded.

"It is obvious to us that you have lied repeatedly and broken so many rules that I have lost count. Not only are you not allowed to have a boy in your room with the door closed, you were in the room with a boy and the door was LOCKED!"

Mike stopped and took a deep breath.

"On top of that, you were smoking marijuana! That is illegal and smoking anything at all is bad for you! Especially with your history! And then this boy escapes through the window! Who is he? And why did he not face me like … like the man he is supposed to be!"

Jackie had to think quickly. What did he mean by those last words?

"We know all about this boyfriend of yours", her mother's voice was shrill; Jackie had never seen her so angry.

"What did Andrea tell you?" Jackie's fear had turned to anger. "I'm going to kill that little …."

"You will do no such thing!" Mike was angrier than he had ever been. "I saw the truck in the driveway! That is not the truck of a 17-year old! How old is this boyfriend of yours? Why are you hiding things from us?"

Jackie looked from one parent to another. She said nothing.

"You are 17 years old, Jackie! You are still a child! How old is this person and what is his name? Are you ashamed to tell us? And are you having sex with him?"

The realization of this made Deb sit down on the only available chair in the room. Mike also needed to sit down but there was nowhere else for him to sit than on Jackie's bed. Jackie immediately moved out of reach.

"For Pete's sake, Jackie, I'm not going to touch you!"

"Okay, okay" Jackie knew she was in big trouble and that she had to tell them the truth.

"His name is Chase. He's twenty I think … no, Dad, please don't look at me like that!" Jackie was crying now. "I met him, well that doesn't matter… He's Charlotte's brother … You know Charlotte, right? She's in my class. Anyway, he's a really nice guy…."

She didn't know what else to say.

Her mother was thinking fast. What if she, they, were having sex? The thought of that made her feel light-headed.

"Jackie, we need to talk about stuff, and maybe you don't want your father to be part of this conversation…."

"Hang on a minute, Deb, what shouldn't I hear?" As the words left his mouth he realized what the talk was going to be about. He really didn't want to be a part of that and he got up quickly.

"You have not heard the end of this …" he muttered as he left the room.

Deb sat quietly for a moment; this was a conversation she really didn't want to have with her 17-year old daughter. But as she thought about it, she knew that it was actually a pretty normal mother–daughter thing.

"Jackie, you have to be honest with me. This is important. Are you having sex with this person?"

Jackie looked at her Mom; her face was red and she appeared to be thinking what to say next.

"It's okay, honey, I'm not mad. If you are having sex I need to know that you're safe…." Deb's managed to keep her voice calm.

Jackie nodded her head. Her face was covered by her long brown hair.

"Phew. Okay." Deb was not sure where to go next….

"Are you being safe? Like … um … are you on birth control? Are you using condoms?"

"Mmmoooommmmm …" Jackie thought she was going to die of embarrassment.

"Seriously, Jackie. We have to talk about this. I know you think you're grown up enough to take care of things, but I just need to hear that you are in fact taking care of things!"

It felt like a trick question to the teenager. Chase had told her that he had an allergic reaction to condoms. She was too scared to argue with him and anyway, because of her cancer, she couldn't get pregnant. She always tried not to think about the cancer but here was a silver lining!

"Mom, I had cancer remember? I can't get pregnant!"

Deb groaned.

"Honey, they removed just the left ovary and the one you have left is working just fine! You get your period every month, right?"

Jackie nodded but a small flutter of fear started in her stomach.

"And you can get an infection from unprotected sex! Do you know that this guy is …. clean? I mean, do you know where he's been and with who? Jackie! He's older than you and I bet way more experienced."

Her mother's words made the flutter in her stomach turn into a loud drumbeat. She didn't really know Chase all that well, and she didn't really want to have sex with him. But she felt left out because all the other girls, the cool girls, she was friendly with talked about it all the time. So she said 'yes' to him…..

Dr Katz advises:

Establishing a sexual identity is another one of the developmental milestones that need to be met during adolescence, particularly in the later years of this stage. This includes figuring out who one is attracted to, sexual identity (who you choose to partner with), and also beginning to experiment with sexual activity. This is often a flashpoint for parents who conveniently forget what they were like at the same age and what they did, often to their parents' consternation!

Individuals who have been treated for cancer often do not know if the treatment has impacted on their fertility and may assume that they cannot conceive, or in the case of males, cannot get someone pregnant. Information about this at the time of diagnosis or treatment may be forgotten or not heard at a time of crisis. This can lead to an unplanned or unwanted pregnancy that will change the course of someone's life.

The other concern about unprotected sexual activity is the risk of getting a sexually transmitted infection (STI) that can have long term-consequences for reproductive and general health. Women often do not have any signs of having a STI and if this is not treated, may result in a serious pelvic infection. Men usually have symptoms of infection and so may go for treatment.

As she thought more about this, Jackie started to cry. Deb reached over and hugged her and for the first time in a very long time, Deb felt needed by her daughter.

"We've only done it once or twice!" Jackie sobbed as she told her mother the whole story of her and Chase. "I didn't really want to do it…." She was crying so hard that she started hiccupping.

As Deb patted her back, she was grateful that Mike had not heard what Jackie had said; he would have been so angry and ready to deal with this Chase person, probably physically. Deb was thinking about what needed to happen next. Certainly a visit to the oncologist to talk about Jackie's fertility, a visit to Dr Brandon to discuss contraception, and a real mother–daughter talk about relationships. It felt to Deb that they had crossed a line in their relationship; Jackie wasn't a little girl anymore but she still needed her mother. Despite the drama of what had happened, perhaps this is what they needed to draw closer together; she was ready for whatever came next.

Conclusion

Adolescence is a time of rapid emotional and physical growth. Parents are often not prepared for the emotional changes that occur, not only for their child but also for the parent–child relationship. This normal event is even more challenging when a child has had cancer or is being treated for cancer. Parents often become more- and even over-protective, and this results in conflict with an adolescent who is changing as part of growing up. There is a delicate balance to looking out for one's child and giving them enough leeway to develop and mature.

Reflective Questions

After reading this story:

- What could the parents in this story done to maintain their relationship with their daughter when her behavior changed?
- How can parents manage their own anxiety when adolescent children start 'acting out'?
- What can parents do when they find out or think that their adolescent child has become sexually active?
- Adolescents naturally think they are invincible; how can parents support their independence while also trying to keep them safe?

9

KEY TASKS FOR YOUNG ADULTS

"I NEED TO MAKE MY OWN WAY AND CREATE MY OWN FAMILY"

Nancy was 24 years old when she was diagnosed with cervical cancer. At the time she was living with her boyfriend James; she noticed some bleeding after sexual intercourse but ignored it. When it happened again a week later, she went to the clinic near their apartment where she saw a nurse practitioner. When questioned about the last time she had a Pap test, Nancy couldn't remember. The nurse practitioner did one immediately and told Nancy that she could expect the results in about a week. Nancy wasn't particularly worried; she told herself that no one in her family had a history of cancer and anyway, bleeding after sex could happen for a lot of reasons.

The phone call came five days later. The nurse practitioner told her that there were some abnormal cells found from the Pap test and that she needed to see a gynecologist. This made Nancy very anxious and when she told James about this, he said she was being hysterical. Things were not going well in their relationship and his attitude to this angered her. She talked to her Mom about this one weekend. Nancy's mother, Marion, had recently retired from her job as manager of a bank. She had been

DOI: 10.4324/9781003242680-9

widowed for many years; Nancy's father had died of a catastrophic heart attack when Nancy was three years old. Marion regarded Nancy as her best friend and wanted to know everything that was going on in Nancy's life.

Nancy saw the gynecologist who wanted to do more tests and now Nancy was really worried. Within two weeks she heard the words that would change her life forever: "Nancy, you have cervical cancer. We think we caught this early, but you are going to have to have surgery to remove your cervix."

Nancy didn't hear the rest of what she was told. She did what the gynecologist told her to do; she had the surgery and stayed with her mom to recover. The surgery removed her cervix and some of the tissues nearby; Nancy did not ask questions of the medical team, preferring to hope that they knew what was best. She really didn't know much about what the treatment meant beyond recovering from the surgery. Her thoughts were focused elsewhere, mostly on her relationship with James.

James didn't visit her and when she called him late one night, there was loud music in the background and what sounded like womens' laughter. Another time when she called him, a woman answered his phone and he was evasive when she asked him who that person was. Nancy's mother didn't like James very much but had always held her tongue when Nancy complained about him. Now that Nancy had talked about how she felt he was treating her, Marion felt this gave her permission to raise her doubts about him.

"Nancy, is he really the right person for you? I don't mean to pry, but he doesn't seem to be treating you very well at all".

Nancy sighed. She was upset about the lack of attention from him and in truth, he had not taken any of this seriously. He often told her she was making a fuss or overthinking things when he should have supported her. Now that her surgery was over and she was feeling better, she had started to think more about the cancer and what it meant.

"I know Mom …" her voice was sad as she told her mother what she had been thinking. "We've been together since I was 19, that's a long time. The lease on the apartment is in my name but he's not going to want to leave. It's going to be a mess if I tell him he has to go…"

"It sounds to me like you've already made up your mind, honey", Marion could not hide the relief in her voice; she was happy that Nancy had come to the realization that her relationship with James was at an end.

A week later Nancy told James that he had to move out. She thought he would put up a fight but he packed his stuff and left quietly. She heard from a friend that he had moved in with another woman soon after they broke up. Nancy was surprised that this news didn't upset her. She was back at work after six weeks of sick leave at the law firm where she was a legal secretary and she found out that she loved living alone. Despite encouragement from her friends and even the lawyer she worked for, she didn't want to date. She didn't feel ready to even think about starting another relationship. She was happy to see her mother every weekend and they went to the movies or out for dinner on Saturday nights. She saw her girlfriends for happy hour once a week and on the other nights, she was happy to be alone in her apartment.

Dr Katz advises:

The years between 19 and 35 are regarded as young adulthood and with this wide age range, the developmental tasks are somewhat different for those at the younger and older ends of the range. At the younger end, early young adults start to engage in relationships that are sexual and many relationships tend to not last a long time. These younger adults are entering college and over time as they reach their late 20s, may have chosen a career path. At the other end of the age range, older young adults may be in a committed relationship with a life partner; they may have one or more children and are established in their careers.

Cancer threatens an individual's ability to establish long-lasting relationships that are emotionally and sexually mature and hopefully committed as well. This commitment should also be present when illness occurs; the partner should be supportive both emotionally and practically. This may mean taking over household tasks, becoming a care giver when necessary, and always providing the support that the person with cancer needs.

Three years later the COVID pandemic happened; the law office closed and Nancy had to work from home. She missed going to the office where there were people to talk to and a staff lounge where she ate lunch with the other legal secretaries. She couldn't see her mom who was in her early 60s and at risk of getting infected, but they talked on the phone most days. Happy hour with her friends no longer happened because the bars were closed. Her friends tried to meet up on Zoom once a week, but it was not the same. She was afraid to go out for a walk because of her cancer history; she avoided contact with the public and ordered groceries online for delivery. She was lonely and as the pandemic stretched on, she grew even lonelier and depressed.

One night on the weekly Zoom call with her friends, Nancy admitted to them that she was not doing well. Poppy, her closest friend, asked if this had to do with the cancer; Nancy quickly assured them that she was fine cancer-wise but she was lonely and a little bored. The change in her daily life was really affecting her and she could see no end in sight.

"Me too!" said Merle and then the rest of the group added that they too were feeling down.

"So how are the rest of you handling this?" Nancy asked. She was surprised that all of them responded with the exception of Poppy.

"I'm drinking!" said Amy and they all laughed.

"Ice cream!" shouted Merle over the laughter.

"I've tried both", said Poppy, "Neither worked but I think I found something that does!"

The three of them waited to hear what Poppy had discovered.

"I rejoined that dating app I was on last year!" Poppy sounded pleased with herself. "I tell you, ladies, I am having the time of my life! There are so many cute guys out there and it's super easy to chat online or on the phone. No getting all dressed up and waiting at the bar like a loser until someone shows up! I do put on some mascara and concealer but that's it. Nice top and pajama bottoms, all in the comfort of my home!"

The others peppered her with questions and Nancy was intrigued; she had not dated since she was 19 when she met James and even though the relationship did not end well, maybe it was time….

That weekend she took a photo of herself; it took a dozen tries to get one that she was happy with but finally she had one that was not too bad. Before she lost her nerve she posted her photo and profile on the website that Poppy used. To her surprise there were five responses to her profile by Monday morning. She read through the men's profiles carefully and disregarded two of them immediately because there were spelling errors in their message to her. Any man who did not check their spelling was not going to be interesting to her, she thought. When she told Poppy, her friend laughed.

"Just because a guy can't spell doesn't mean much", Poppy told her but Nancy insisted that this meant he was lazy.

"Okay then, my friend, maybe you'll find a teacher or a writer!"

She responded to the other three men who had messaged her and decided that one of them was interesting. His name was Robert and he was a musician; his message to her was written after midnight and he explained that he had been on a Zoom session with some other musicians till late. The messages flew back and forth for the next few days and finally, he asked Nancy if they could talk on the phone.

Nancy told her mother about this on one of their calls. Marion was shocked and had a long list of concerns that she shared with her daughter: Was this safe and who was this person? What if he wasn't who he said he was? Did she intend to meet him in person and how could this be safe with COVID around?

"Mom, it's oaky. We're just talking on the phone! I'm not going to meet him in person just yet! Please don't ruin this for me! It's been a long time since I was even interested is dating anyone and I know what I'm doing!" She sounded braver than she felt; she was nervous to meet a man after this time.

Dr Katz advises:

There are always generational differences when it comes to opinions about dating. For those now in their 60s, dating was often more formal, with the man asking the woman to go to dinner and/or a movie for their first date. That generation is the generation of 'free love' and the birth control pill! But as a person matures, they often become more conservative and forget what they did in the past. Dating is more egalitarian for young adults today, and many couples meet through a dating site.

In many ways this is much safer than meeting at a bar or concert. Online dating allows for time and space to get to know each other before meeting in person. Of course there are also dating sites that are used primarily for a 'hook-up', a 21st-century phenomenon where people meet up purely for sex.

Nancy and Robert talked on the phone later that week. To her surprise, the call lasted almost two hours. He was so interesting to talk to and he seemed so interested in her! This was so different from James who seemed to have lost interest in her over time. Robert asked a lot of questions about her work, her family, her hobbies (she didn't have any!), and her taste in music. It had been a very long time since anyone had given her this much attention and she found that she liked talking about herself!

When she realized how much time had passed, she suggested that they talk again. She had hardly had the chance to ask him about his own life but she had to get up early to finish working on something for one of the partners that had an upcoming deadline. Robert was eager to talk to her again so they made arrangements to talk the next evening. Nancy was worried about if and when she should tell him about her cancer history. It seemed like ages ago that she was treated and despite going every six months for follow-up tests and visits to the oncologist, she didn't think about it much at all. The doctor seemed pretty confident that she was cured and Nancy took her at her word.

Soon they were talking every night, sometimes into the early hours of the morning. After another two weeks and many phone calls, Nancy decided that she had to tell him about the cancer. She was not sure how to go about it; how did one introduce such a heavy topic? She didn't know who to ask for advice so she searched on the internet to see if there was a correct way to do this. She came up empty; there was nothing of use to her online. One night they were talking about their family and Robert mentioned quite casually that his father was being treated for prostate cancer. Nancy saw this as an opportunity to tell him but she was nervous. What if this meant the end of their fledgling relationship?

"Um, Rob… I have something to tell you…."

"Okay, shoot … I'm listening…."

"Um, three years ago I was diagnosed with cervical cancer…."

There was a pause and Robert took a breath. Nancy was preparing herself for rejection and she held her breath.

"Oh, I'm sorry … hang on, is that even the right thing to say?" Robert sounded flustered. "I mean that's a rotten thing to have…. How old were you? Oh, I didn't mean to say that…. Maybe I should just stop and let you say something before I mess this up completely!"

Nancy couldn't help laughing. She was not sure what she expected him to say but his response struck her as almost funny.

"It's okay, Rob. I wasn't sure how to tell you, or even when I should … but I want to be honest with you. If this is a deal breaker for you, then we can go on with our life and no hard feelings. I just don't think it's fair to not be honest with you about my past. You know about James my ex, and his response to my diagnosis was the reason for us breaking up…."

"Yeah, I wondered why you broke up with him…."

Nancy really didn't want to talk about James so she changed the subject.

"What do you want to know about the cancer…. I'll answer any questions you have…."

Dr Katz advises:

There is no 'perfect' or 'right' time to tell someone about a cancer history. Everyone is different and the nature of the relationship is unique to the people involved. It is difficult for both the person disclosing as well as the person hearing this. How does one tell or respond?

The person hearing this may feel a bit like a deer caught in the headlights. What is the right thing to say? What is the absolute wrong thing to say? What if your response makes the other person feel bad? How do you show interest in hearing more without being intrusive? This likely feels like a minefield.

A question such as: "Are you okay to tell me more about how this affected you"? shows interest but allows the person who has had cancer to control the amount of detail they provide. An empathetic statement is also appropriate: "That must have been tough…."

The most important thing is to be authentic in response as well as avoiding statements such as "You don't look like someone who had cancer" or platitudes such as "But you look so great"!

After a further couple of weeks, they started to schedule video calls and Nancy was pleased to see that his profile picture was no different from his appearance in real life. He was smart, had a good sense of humor, and most of all, he was not pressuring her to meet in person. She was nervous about being in public because of the COVID pandemic and she also didn't feel ready to take the relationship to the 'next level' where it could become physical.

Nancy had avoided telling her mother anything about Robert. Marion's initial response to Nancy meeting someone online irritated Nancy. If her mother was going to continue being suspicious and negative, there was no point in sharing anything about their calls and video chats. Marion asked constantly about her life and Nancy usually gave vague answers. That did not stop Marion.

"This is not a good time to be dating, Nancy", she remarked one evening on their regular phone call. "With COVID and…."

"I know, Mom! You don't to have to keep reminding me! I'm 27 and life is passing me by!"

Marion immediately stopped talking; she heard the pain in Nancy's voice and felt guilty. She was lonely too and wished that she could see Nancy instead of the phone calls that were not satisfying. Nancy often sounded like she had better things to do than talk to her mother. Was it possible that she was indeed dating? She had been evasive when Marion asked her questions about what she was doing.

"Nancy, are you still seeing that guy you met on the computer?"

Nancy didn't bother to correct her mother; she was not seeing anyone ON the computer! But she needed to be careful how she answered the question about Robert.

"There's someone that I've talked to a couple of times…."

"Is it the same chap you talked about before? That musician? Nancy, you can do better than that! He will never earn a living and there are always going to be girls hanging around … what do you call them? Oh yes, groupies".

Nancy felt her temper rising. Before she said something that she might regret, she told her mother she had to go. She felt badly for her Mom. She had been alone for so long, more than 20 years now, and she had always depended on Nancy for company. And now with the COVID pandemic, she was really alone. Nancy knew that her mother's questions and assumptions were in part a response to her loneliness and missing Nancy's company, but Nancy had a right to a life of her own.

Over the next month, Nancy and Robert met once a week at a park that had circles painted on the grass to encourage social distancing. She was very nervous the first time they met, but soon relaxed as they started to talk. Robert's eyes were the most beautiful green and they grew even greener when he smiled. She had pinned her dirty blond hair into a bun and Robert reached across to move some hair that had fallen across her face. She felt a spark as he did that and in an instant, she realized that she wanted more of him and the relationship.

As COVID case numbers decreased over the following months, Nancy felt more confident about seeing him. And the social distancing seemed less and less important. Soon she and Robert were seeing each other almost every day and he stayed over three or four times a week. They had talked about their future and it involved a wedding and children, at least that's what Robert wanted. Nancy was not sure about the children part; she was unsure about her fertility and fears about the cancer's impact on that now kept her up at night. Would she be able to get pregnant? She was 28 now and while her biological clock was not exactly ticking, she was afraid that a pregnancy could make the cancer come back. And what if her body couldn't carry a pregnancy for the full nine months? She didn't tell Robert what she was thinking and evaded any discussions about this.

Dr Katz advises:

Cancer survivors often don't remember all the information they were given at the time of diagnosis or during treatment. There is a LOT to take in and over time, the information fades into the background. This is especially true for young adults who have been given information about the treatment's effects on future fertility. They may not have given much thought to having children at the time of their treatment. When the time comes that they are considering having a family, they are unsure about how their cancer and/or its treatment may impact on this.

Asking for detailed information about any treatment for the cancer – surgery, radiation, chemotherapy and other medications – and having a discussion about the potential impacts these on fertility is important. This information should be provided by the treating oncologist. If treatment confers a risk to fertility, patients should be offered the opportunity to see a fertility specialist and offered sperm or eggs/embryos freezing. This may be possible before treatment starts, but in some instances, treatment needs to start immediately and a delay is not possible. Fertility status can be assessed by a fertility specialist after treatment is over and when the person wants to start a family. For men, a semen analysis will assess the presence and quality of sperm. For women, blood tests to measure hormones and/or ultrasound can be used to assess fertility; the presence of menstrual periods is not an accurate estimate of fertility.

A few months passed; Robert had moved in with Nancy and her apartment was filled with music when Robert was home. She initially thought that this would disturb her work, but she found that she loved it. Once both of them had been vaccinated against COVID they started seeing friends more frequently; her girlfriends loved Robert and she got on well with his musician buddies. They avoided talking about having children because any mention of this led to arguments. The last time they fought about this Robert challenged Nancy about her fears.

"Why don't you just go and see someone who can help you figure out if pregnancy is possible?"

Nancy had stared at him with tears in her eyes. She knew that her avoidance was irrational but she couldn't help herself. What if she could never get pregnant? Or perhaps even worse, what if the surgery she had made carrying a pregnancy the full nine months impossible? What if she miscarried? Robert really wanted to have a family and she was scared that if they knew for sure that this was not possible, would he leave her? And then there was the question of money.

Robert didn't earn much as a musician before the pandemic and when any kind of work dried up because of the pandemic, he lived off his savings. Nancy's job paid fairly well, but she was now supporting the two of them and things were tight financially. Fertility treatments were expensive, she knew that because one of her colleagues at work had gone through it and talked about the expense. The simple truth was that they could not afford it but talking about money with Robert was a problem; he felt guilty about depending on Nancy for almost everything and he got upset at any mention of this.

And then there was her mother. Marion had still not accepted their relationship. Because of COVID Nancy had a good excuse to not see her, but now as things were getting back to something like normal, the distance between them was more obvious. Whereas before Robert, Nancy would have felt comfortable asking her mother for a loan, there was no way she was going to do that now. The irony was that Marion would have loved having a grandchild or two, but Nancy would not ask her for money now. Marion talked about this is a joking way but Nancy could tell that she was serious. Once she even suggested to her daughter that perhaps this was Robert's fault; Nancy burst out laughing at the irony. If only Marion knew that it was Nancy who was afraid of getting pregnant and Robert was just fine.

Dr Katz advises:

The topic of pregnancy is a delicate one and parents need to tiptoe around the subject in most instances. This is a very private issue and any questions may be seen as intrusive. Questions when a couple is experiencing infertility can also be hurtful. Parents will be informed, usually with great joy, when the couple wants to disclose the happy event.

Cancer treatment-related infertility is quite common, especially for those who have been treated with chemotherapy or radiation to the pelvis. Chemotherapy attacks rapidly dividing cells, like cancer cells, but also the ovaries and testicles in some cases, depending on the specific chemotherapy used. While men produce sperm from puberty till death, women are born with all the eggs they will ever have. Chemotherapy may stop the production of eggs permanently or cause early menopause. Radiation to the pelvis in women may impact on the ability of the uterus to expand during pregnancy. And surgery to the reproductive organs may have a significant impact on sperm production as well as the ability to conceive and carry a pregnancy. Individuals diagnosed with cancer who are of child-bearing age should be offered fertility preservation before treatment starts. This is not always possible if treatment needs to start immediately, but banking sperm can be done a few days before the start of treatment. The situation is more complicated for women who need medication to stimulate the ovaries to produce eggs that are then frozen; generally a delay in starting treatment for about two weeks is needed for this.

Robert grew increasingly frustrated as Nancy procrastinated and delayed and avoided making an appointment at the fertility clinic. He tried talking to her but she responded with annoyance.

"I can't talk about this now" was her usual reply when he asked about this.

"Is it the money?" he asked, "I'll find a full-time job and we can save my earnings...."

"It's not the damn money, Robert!"

"Then what is it? It's been months and you won't talk about it and you won't make an appointment! Please tell me what your reluctance is!"

"I do. Not. Want. To. Have. Children!" Nancy was surprised by the anger in her voice.

"What? I mean, you never said...." He was shocked at her outburst.

"I mean ... I.... Robert! What if I can't have children?"

This was something completely different from not wanting to have children and Robert reached out and pulled her toward him.

"Nancy, love, this is something different.... You don't know you can't have kids.... If you, I mean we, go to the fertility clinic at least we'll know ...." Robert was almost begging her.

Her voice was muffled because she was crying into his shirt.

"Okay, okay. I'll go".

Once the appointment was made, Nancy could not back down, although she tried. Each time she wanted to cancel the appointment, Robert reminded her that they were only going to get information and nothing more. What he didn't tell her was that he had started applying for jobs so that if they decided to go ahead with investigations and treatment, there would be money to cover at least part of the bills. The morning of the appointment Nancy felt nauseous and refused to get out of bed. Robert laughed at her and carried her into the bathroom.

"You want me to throw you in the shower? Or maybe get in there with you?"

Nancy couldn't help but laugh; she was completely aware that she was being immature and so she showered, got dressed and was waiting for Robert when he emerged from their bedroom, his hair wet and his face shiny. As they walked to the car, he put his arm around her and kissed the top of her head. She could tell he was excited and she tried to keep her anxiety in check.

The fertility clinic was very fancy and Robert felt a little intimidated. He did not have much experience with medical institutions and he felt his excitement disappear. No wonder people say these treatments cost a lot! They didn't have to wait long before being ushered into an office that was furnished all in white, following the color scheme of the waiting room. There were colorful paintings on the wall and a large computer monitor on the desk. They sat down on the two white leather chairs facing the empty chair across the desk. Nancy reached over to hold Robert's hand; he looked nervous probably because he felt uncomfortable in the surroundings.

The door to the office opened and a young woman rushed in, apologizing as she sat down.

"Sorry I'm late!" She glanced up at a clock on the wall behind Nancy and Robert. "Oh, just 5 minutes! But apologies just the same".

The couple didn't say anything and looked at her expectantly.

"I'm Dr Springer. Nancy, I received the notes from your surgery and I've also talked to the surgeon who operated on you".

Robert sat up straighter in the chair.

"I have some information for you. The surgery you had removed the cervix as you know. This does not affect your chances of getting pregnant…."

Nancy heard Robert exhale.

"But there is an increased risk of miscarriage as the uterus grows. From the perspective of your fertility, our services won't be needed unless you don't get pregnant within a year. You should be under the care of an obstetrician who focuses on high-risk pregnancies once you do get pregnant. Do you have any questions?"

Nancy's mind was going a mile a minute and Robert looked like someone had hit him over the head with a baseball bat.

"Um…. I should follow up with my oncologist?" Nancy was uncertain about what to do next.

"You should be seeing your oncologist regularly and you can certainly talk to them. But if you want to get pregnant now, you should see an OB who deals with high risk pregnancies".

Dr Springer seemed a little irritated that Nancy did not understand what she had just said. She started to get out of her chair as she switched off the computer. The consultation was over.

"Well that was short and sweet", whispered Robert as the doctor left the room.

"Yeah", said Nancy, "I wonder what that is going to cost…."

They walked back to the car, both lost in thought.

"Can we go for a walk and talk about this? I'm not due to be back at work till after lunch. I had no idea how long this would take…." Nancy had not expected the news that they had received from the doctor.

"Sure, let's go to the park. I need to get some coffee on the way".

The park was quiet at this time of day; in the distance they could hear the laughter of children playing on the swings so they walked a little further along the path. When all they could hear was the birds singing in the trees they stopped and sat on a bench.

"What are you thinking, Nancy?"

Robert's voice was soft and non-committal. He was scared that if he showed any enthusiasm, Nancy would shut him down.

"I'm not sure what I'm thinking. I guess I should be happy that we don't need to start with the fertility stuff, but I'm still scared. That doctor said I was high-risk…."

"She said that any pregnancy would be a high-risk pregnancy, not that you were high risk", Robert tried to correct her.

"I KNOW that, Robert!" Nancy was quick to get irritated. "I just used the wrong term, that's all!"

She gazed across the green field as if there was something fascinating happening in the distance.

"Okay, I'm sorry. I just thought that is was good news…."

"I guess so…" Nancy replied, "So what do we do now?"

"Well, I guess we could go home and …."

He didn't finish the sentence; Nancy glared at him. How did he think that sex was going to relieve her anxiety?

"I was just trying to be funny … but I guess the timing isn't right".

Nancy didn't answer. She was deep in thought, wondering what she should do next. She loved Robert and wanted to spend the rest of her life with him. But she was still not sure about having children. Would this be a deal breaker, or could they find a compromise, if there even was one? So many questions, she thought to herself, and no easy answers.

Conclusion

Young adulthood is a time when many decisions have to be made, most of them big decisions with no easy answers. This is a stage when serious relationships should be cemented and plans made for having children, or not. Young adults at the lower end of the age range may be at college or at the beginning of their career. Those at the older end should be well on their way to being established in their career and life plans. But cancer interrupts the achievement of many of these life plans and goals. The parent(s) and partner of the individual with cancer must be careful to not put pressure or interfere in how the cancer survivor attempts to engage in life again; this helps to avoid stressors in the relationship when support is needed.

Reflective Questions

After reading this story:

- How as a parent do you manage to keep quiet when you know your young adult child is in a bad relationship?
- What advice would you give to a young adult about when and how to disclose a cancer history?
- How can the partner of a young adult with cancer support their partner while at the same being able to express their own feelings about building a family?
- How could the fertility specialist have provided more supportive care to this young couple?

10

WHERE TO FIND HELP

"WHO AND WHAT CAN WE TRUST"?

Jonathan is a civil engineer who works for his father Norman, who is the owner of a large and successful construction company. Jonathan loves his work; as a young boy he imagined himself in a yellow hard hat, pushing mounds of dirt from the seat of a front-end loader. His father encouraged him to get an engineering degree; it was always Norman's wish to have his son in the business. Jonathan is a 'hands on' kind of guy. He can often be found on a work site, a yellow hard hat on his head, walking around and chatting to the guys pouring concrete or erecting scaffolding.

Jonathan has lived at home ever since he graduated. At 34 years old, he sees nothing wrong in living with his parents despite almost constant teasing from his sister Sylvie, who is two years younger than him. Sylvie is a physiotherapist and is married to her college boyfriend Matt. She could not wait to leave home and has never returned to the family home after college. She and Matt live a five-minute walk from her parents and are often to be found there, hanging out on the deck or having dinner with her parents and Jonathan.

DOI: 10.4324/9781003242680-10

Their mother, Adele, is the glue that keeps them so close. A retired nurse, she is the quintessential caregiver who cooks and entertains and has her finger on the pulse of what is happening with her grown children. She has always welcomed their friends, and the friends of their friends, and there is almost always a full cookie jar on the kitchen counter. Adele retired five years ago; she had back troubles from her years at the bedside and she was tired. Nursing had become more difficult after her hospital was bought out by a large health care company, and every day seemed more of a battle than a joy. There were days when she missed it, but Sylvie's stories about her career kept her emotionally satisfied, without the back pain!

One day about a month before, Jonathan noticed some bleeding on the toilet tissue after a bowel movement. He was not concerned but it happened about three days later and this time there was blood in the toilet bowl, not just on the tissue. He mentioned it to Sylvie who told him that this was not something to ignore and that he needed to see a doctor. Like many young men his age, Jonathan did not have a doctor; he went to an Urgent Care facility on the odd occasion that he hurt himself on the job site and once when he had a STI. He threatened Sylvie that if she told either of their parents, he would never talk to her again.

Three days later, Sylvie texted him to say that she had talked to one of the doctors at the hospital where she worked. She made an appointment for Jonathan to see this doctor, a gastroenterologist, and that he had to go to the appointment, no ifs, ands, or buts. This time she threatened him that if he did not go to the appointment, she would never talk to him again. She offered to go with him but he was firm in his insistence that he didn't need her to be there.

"Seriously, Sylvie? I'm your big brother, remember?"

Sylvie shook her head. He had never asked for her help for anything. But she was a physio and could try and help him understand what the GI doctor told him. She decided not to argue with him but couldn't resist a parting shot: "Okay but remember who got you the appointment...."

Jonathan went to the appointment with the doctor. He was okay in a distant and professional way. Dr Blackburn told Jonathan that he needed to have a digital rectal exam to start with, followed by some other more invasive tests.

"Like a digital rectal exam is not invasive"! Jonathan thought to himself.

The examination did not take long.

"I can feel something about an inch past the anus", Dr Blackburn said, his voice not showing any alarm. You're going to need a CT and MRI and possibly a PET scan".

Jonathan heard the last part of what the doctor said. He dressed quickly, thanked the doctor and walked to his car where he sat for a while before leaving the parking garage. He missed the turnoff to his office and drove for about ten miles before realizing that he was nowhere near when he was supposed to be. He pulled over to the shoulder of the road and sat with his head on the steering wheel. What was he going to do now, he thought, this was not supposed to happen to someone his age!

Dr Katz advises:

Believing that cancer only happens to older adults, young adults may ignore signs that something is not right. Rectal bleeding is never something that should be ignored. It may be haemorrhoids or a fissure, but this needs medical attention. Ignoring symptoms like this can lead to a delay in diagnosis, resulting in cancer being found at a later stage. This may mean a poor prognosis with more intense treatment or even spread to other parts of the body. When this happens, cure is no longer possible and control of the cancer is the best that can be hoped for.

Because cancer is rare in younger people, some young adults might see a health care provider who may assume that the person does not have cancer because of their age, not order diagnostic tests, and thus a cancer diagnosis is missed or delayed. This will have the same end result as the individual ignoring symptoms and delaying care.

Sylvie asked him about the appointment; he knew she was going to ask, and he had prepared a response.

"Um, he said that I need to have more tests…."

"Tests for what? Don't lie to me, Jonathan! If he found something, I need to know! Mom and Dad too! You can't hide stuff from us!"

It sounded like she was going to cry and Jonathan felt bad. He loved his sister so much and was proud of her career choice.

"Okay, okay…" Jonathan was not sure how he was going to get the words out.

"He said he felt something in my…" Now he was on the verge of tears.

"What??? Just tell me!!! Nothing could be worse than what I am imagining…"

Jonathan took a deep breath. "Syl, he said I had a lesion or something in my….ugh…anus! Is that even a thing?"

Sylvie started to cry, and she tried to get some control over her voice.

"Okay, okay, let me think for a minute…"

"How am I going to tell Mom and Dad? This is going to kill them…."

"Hang on", Sylvie said. Jonathan heard her blowing her nose. "Okay, we'll do this together. What exactly did the doctor say?"

Jonathan was not sure. All he remembered was the words "lesion" and "anus" and "tests".

"Okay – so nothing is certain, at least for now. We, I mean, you will tell them when you know for sure. Okay?" Sylvie knew they were just buying time but that would allow her to find out more about this.

Jonathan had a CT scan and a MRI. He had been referred to a surgeon, a cancer surgeon, at the hospital where Sylvie worked. She sat with him while he waited to have the tests and she was there when they were finished. He didn't know how she got time off from her shift but he was grateful that she was there. He was terrified.

Later that week, he and Sylvie met with the surgeon. Dr Danan was young, about their age, and friendly. He explained everything to them; Jonathan would need surgery but the lesion was small so he would not need to have an ostomy. Jonathan felt all the blood drain from his face. Ostomy? He remembered the grandfather of one of his friends when he was a teenager who had a 'poop bag'. They used to laugh at the old guy who often smelled really bad. A wave of shame passed through him; how horrible they were to the man. He might also need chemotherapy and radiation but that would be determined by what was found when the lesion was removed.

Jonathan's head swam and he felt nauseous. This was happening too fast and he was not prepared for this. And then there was the need to tell his parents. He imagined his mother's face and how she would fight back tears by biting her lip until it bled. His father would straighten his shoulders and look across the room, as if he was examining a speck of paint on the wrong place on the wall.

He told his parents the next day. It was almost exactly as he had imagined, except for the part where tears ran down his father's face. His mother said nothing and he could see a muscle on the side of her face twitching. Sylvie sat next to him, squeezing his hand while he talked. He told them that he needed surgery and that was all he knew for sure. The surgery was scheduled for later that month.

"I need to get out of here, Syl", he whispered to his sister. "Can you stay with them for a bit and answer any questions they have?"

Sylvie nodded her head. "Mom, Dad ... Jonathan needs some space right now. I'll stick around if you need to ask anything but then I have to leave too. Matt is home and I haven't seen much of him this week". Norman and Adele both nodded but Sylvie was not sure they had heard. The three of them sat in silence for a while and then Sylvie got up, kissed them both, and went home.

The next morning Jonathan's mother knocked on his door, waking him from a restless sleep.

"Jonathan, it's Mom. I've been researching this thing that you have and here's what you need to do!"

Jonathan sat up in bed. His head was fuzzy and he could barely open his eyes.

"Mom, whoa ... hold on a second! What are you talking about? What do you mean?"

"I couldn't sleep last night and so I started looking up this stuff on the internet and I found this place where you can get stuff ... um, herbs and stuff that will help you to avoid surgery. Isn't that great?"

Jonathan groaned. He had a feeling that this was going to happen. His mother, despite being trained as a nurse, had a strong belief in herbs and things that were 'natural'.

Dr Katz advises:

A cancer diagnosis causes a loss of control in many different aspects of daily life. In an attempt to regain some semblance of control, people often try to find something that they can control as this may reduce their anxiety and fear of the unknown. One way of doing this is to look for 'natural' or unconventional treatments that claim to treat cancer. These include herbs, alkaline or acidic diets, cannabis oil, mega doses of vitamins, Laetrile (apricot pits), and essential oils. There are also claims that coffee or water enemas, muscle strength training (applied kinesiology), ozone therapy, or positive thinking can cure cancer.

None of these so-called 'cures' have been tested in rigorous clinical trials and many are actually dangerous. It is also known that people who use these 'natural' remedies are more likely to refuse some medical treatments that then leads to poor outcomes. There is no conspiracy in traditional medical care to withhold information about 'natural' treatments. Some complementary therapies can be helpful while people undergo treatment, however they should not replace traditional treatments such as radiation, chemotherapy, or surgery.

Many patients or their family members don't know that some of the medical treatments used to treat cancer are derived from plants. For example, one chemotherapy agent used to treat breast cancer, called a taxane, is derived from the yew tree. If a 'natural' treatment is thought to be useful in cancer care, it will be tested in clinical trials to ensure that it is both safe and effective.

Jonathan called his sister and told her what their mother was doing. Now it was Sylvie's turn to groan. She of course knew that their mother was into this natural stuff, and for the most part it was harmless. When Adele got a migraine, she used essential oils instead of pain medication. She lay in a dark room until the pain passed and the family thought that merely lying in the dark was probably more helpful than the smelly oils. But Jonathan's cancer was another matter.

"Okay, I'll talk to her", replied Sylvie with a sigh. "But I know she's not going to listen to me. She'll say something about how PTs now are over-educated and some other nonsense about not listening to people who actually KNOW about this…. It's so frustrating!"

"Thanks, Syl. I'm so tired of thinking about this all the damn time. I just wish the surgery was over and I could get on with my life".

Sylvie said nothing; she was worried that his life would never be the same. Despite her training as a PT, she did not know much about oncology. The hospital where she worked didn't even have an oncology unit; there was a cancer center that was part of the medical complex where her hospital was located but they were separate buildings and she didn't know anyone who worked there.

Later that day, Adele visited Jonathan at his office. It was not unusual for her to drop in to see him, after all it was her husband's construction company and she felt she had a right to visit. Jonathan was immersed in reviewing plans for a new condo development and startled when the door opened. He was irritated that she had not knocked but the look on her face stopped him from saying anything.

"Mom, you look like you've seen a ghost! Do I look weird?"

His attempt at humor fell flat. Adele had a folder with papers in it, pieces torn out of newspapers and magazines and sheets of paper that she had printed off the internet.

"Jonathan! Look what I found! There's this doctor in ... I forget where, oh yes, now I remember ... Boston ... but anyway he says he can treat cancer with these injections of this stuff that doesn't harm healthy tissues! There are a bunch of testimonials from patients who avoided surgery and toxic chemotherapy because of him. He was trained at Harvard and has a long list of degrees! He looks legit and his office is not so far away.... I looked it up and he's just outside Boston, and it's just a one-hour flight from here!"

Jonathan put his head on his desk. He was frustrated and sad and angry. Why was she wasting her time with this? She was a NURSE! Or at least she had been one for years before she retired. When did her training change to believing this nonsense?

"Mom, please listen to me. I am not going to go and see this quack in Boston! No, don't look at me like that! Why would I believe this rather than the doctor I saw?" Jonathan tried to reason with her, but she wasn't listening.

"Because if you see this doctor that I found on the internet, you don't need to have the surgery and you would be cured!" Adele was persistent.

"And how do you know that he is not a quack? A snake oil salesman who will take my money and then when the cancer gets worse, he won't be found? Or he'll claim I did something wrong?"

"But he's from Harvard!!!"

Hearing their raised voices, Norman entered Jonathan's office.

"What on earth is going on here? Adele, the secretaries can hear you down the hall! What are you arguing about"?

Adele opened her mouth to speak but Jonathan started explaining before she could talk.

"Mom is trying to persuade me to see some quack she found on the internet! I am not interested but she won't stop ... please get her out of here. I need to finish reviewing the plans for the condo development and I can't get anything done with her yapping at me!"

The mention of the condo development gave Norman the impetus he needed to get his wife out of Jonathan's office.

"Honey, this condo development is a high priority and Jonathan has to get this done by the end of the day. Why don't you come to my office and we can talk about what you've found?"

Norman ushered his wife into his office and they sat down to talk. Adele told him about this doctor who said he cures cancer with injections. If Adele hadn't been looking at the paper on her lap she would have seen the expression on her husband's face. He was incredulous and also baffled by why she, a nurse, would believe this nonsense.

"Adele, honey ... the doctors here have recommended surgery. We have to trust them. Do you think that if these injections or whatever worked, that the doctors Jonathan has seen wouldn't be using them too?"

Adele glanced at him and then opened her mouth to argue.

"NO. Stop! Adele I cannot listen to any more of this!" Norman's voice was loud and he realized that he could be heard outside the office. "You have to stop this! It is not doing Jonathan any good and it is certainly starting to make me mad. What has got into you? This is not the Adele that I know..."

Dr. Katz advises:
   All medical products such as drugs and devices must get approval from the FDA before they can be used. This approval assures the public that the products are safe and also effective.
   The FDA sends warning letters to companies that claim to have effective treatment(s) that are not approved by the agency. If these companies do not comply with the FDA orders to stop advertising or selling their products, legal action can be taken against them.

If any product claims to treat all kinds of cancers or shrink/kill cancer cells and tumors, this is likely a fraudulent product. Claims that the product is more effective than chemotherapy should also be a warning sign.

People with cancer can have access to new drugs that are under investigation by participating in clinical trials. The cancer team caring for the person with cancer will know about these trials and will often encourage participation if the person is eligible. The National Cancer Institute Clinical Trials website has information for the public on these trials. The website can be accessed at https://www.cancer.gov/about-cancer/treatment/clinical-trials/search. To read more about the FDA's advise on fraudulent claims about cancer treatment visit https://www.fda.gov/consumers/consumer-updates/products-claiming-cure-cancer-are-cruel-deception.

To his surprise, Adele started to cry. He had always regarded her as so strong; nothing could faze her not even the time that Jonathan had fallen out of a tree in their yard and broken three bones. She had scooped him up gently, put him in the backseat of their car and driven slowly to the emergency department, singing to him all the while. Norman had arrived at the ED, sweating and out of breath, to find Jonathan lying on a gurney, his eyes clouded with pain but staring at his mother as she continued to sing to him.

"Adele, honey … tell me what you're thinking … let me in, please. I don't know what to do … our boy…"

He couldn't finish the sentence and put his head in his hands, his face against her shoulder.

This caused Adele to take a deep breath, wipe the tears from her eyes, and turn to comfort him. They sat together, close but yet far from each other, and they talked. Adele told him that she knew how bad this was for Jonathan and that she felt helpless. She had started to search for articles about Jonathan's cancer. Part of her knew that a lot of what she read was probably inaccurate, but she was desperate. This was her son, her first born, and she was terrified. Norman told her that he too was terrified but if he just kept on hoping for the best, then everything would be okay. He tried to take his lead from Jonathan who seemed to be coping.

"I think our boy is in denial", said Adele. "He seems to be calm … he likely gets that from you".

She smiled for the first time in what seemed like weeks.

"I have an idea", Norm's voice was soft. "Let's see if Sylvie can help. Maybe she can talk to one of her doctor colleagues. Or better yet, perhaps she can go to the medical library at the hospital and find some articles in journals".

"Oh, that's a great idea! Why didn't I think about that!"

Adele looked as if a weight had been lifted from her shoulders.

"I'll text her. She gets off at 3 or 3:30 and maybe she can go to the library today!"

Sylvie was happy to go to the library to find out more about the cancer and its treatment. The librarian was friendly and offered to help Sylvie do a search for articles from the library database. There were a LOT of articles and the librarian showed her how to focus her search so that she got more relevant and up to date articles. Usually customers at the library would have to do their own searches but it was almost the end of the day and helping Sylvie was a distraction from what the librarian was doing. She even printed out a pile of articles for Sylvie to take home.

Sylvie was exhausted and decided that she would start reading the articles on the weekend when she did not have to work. But her parents had another idea and as soon as she walked through the door of her house, there was a text from her mom asking what she found. Her husband Matt shook his head as she put on her shoes and walked out the door to take the articles to them. She called him as she walked the short distance to her parents' house, her footsteps slowing when he answered.

"I have to stay there for a while", she told Matt with a sigh, "I don't think they are going to be able to translate all the medical lingo … it's been a while since Mom worked as a nurse … and anyway, I want to know what's in these articles. Why don't you come over? Mom probably has enough for all of us for dinner…"

Matt said he was on his way and before she had walked to the end of the block, she heard him calling for her to wait for him as he ran down the sidewalk.

Jonathan wasn't home when they got to her parents' house. He had called to say he was staying at the office to finish his review of the condo plans. Adele was worried that he would miss dinner, but he reassured her that he had some protein bars in his desk drawer; he wasn't hungry anyway and continuing to work would take his mind off the surgery scheduled in just days.

The four of them, Norman and Adele, Matt and Sylvie, divided the pile of articles and started to read. Norman didn't make it through the first page of the first article.

"This is a foreign language to me, Sylvie! I seriously can't make head or tail of what they're talking about!"

"Me too" added Matt, "This is way beyond my small brain".

Adele was still reading, a highlighter in her hand, that she swiped over words and sentences.

"Mom? Is this helpful?" Sylvie asked. She had found some of the more technical terms difficult to understand. It had been almost a decade since she finished college and anatomy was a topic that she had always struggled with.

"Um, kind of…" replied Adele, the look on her face suggested that what she had read was not really helpful".

"Really? You look a little shocked", interjected Norman. "Honey, I gave up on the first page of the one I read. Tell us truthfully, is this doing any good?" He gestured at the pages on their laps.

"Honestly? This is scaring me!" Adele admitted. "I don't understand most of it and I'm just highlighting the sentences that are confusing!" She had a sheepish smile on her face and Norman kissed her on the cheek.

"If I'm really truthful, what I think I understood was actually terrifying. I don't want to read anymore of this. Sylvie, I'm sorry. You went to so much trouble to get these articles, but they are really scaring me…"

Norman stood up: "That's it, then! Let's put away these darn papers and eat dinner. We'll all feel better with some food in our stomachs. We can then make a plan for where we can find information that we at least understand!"

Dr Katz advises:
    While articles in professional journals present fact-based information, they can be difficult for the lay public to understand. At best they are difficult to read, using technical terms and academic language, and at worst, can frighten the reader with statistics and conclusions

that present upsetting outcomes. If you have the opportunity to read these articles with a health professional who can interpret the language, this may make the content understandable and even helpful. But often these types of articles are difficult for the average health care consumer. It is often not enough to be able to understand what is written, but to truly evaluate the content, you need to be able to critically analyze what the authors have written and this may require an understanding of complex statistics and deep knowledge of the field.

The next time Sylvie was at work, just days before Jonathan's surgery, she consulted the librarian again on her way home. She explained that her family found the journal articles confusing and even frightening and asked the librarian if she had any suggestions that might help them.

"I thought this might happen", the librarian replied. "I do have some suggestions about how to find legitimate and helpful websites that might be a better fit".

"That would be GREAT! I feel really embarrassed that I also found the articles hard to read, and I'm a PT..."

"You may be a PT, but that does not make you an expert in everything", the librarian said with a smile.

"That's for sure. And this is happening to my brother ... it's different when a member of your family is affected!"

The librarian gave Sylvie a document that described how to assess whether a website is legitimate as well as tips for evaluating the information. As Sylvie glanced over the document, she wondered if her mother had even thought of these factors when she was doing her 'research' for information on the internet.

"This is so helpful, thanks so much. I'll try to not bother you again..." she said as she headed for the glass door that led outside.

"It's my pleasure to help, even though I would rather it was under better circumstances. I wish your brother well, and to your family too".

Sylvie went straight to her parents' house and gave her mother the information from the librarian.

"Do you think I'm an idiot?" Adele said as she read the document. "I do know how to search for information!"

"Oh Mom, please don't get angry with me. I'm trying to help, that's all. I didn't know a lot of this, and I've been using the internet since I was 12 years old!"

Dr Katz advises:

While there is a lot of information on the internet, not all websites are created equal. While they may look professional and authentic, this does not mean that they are reliable and present accurate information. According to Dalhousie University in Canada, there are six criteria for assessing websites (https://cdn.dal.ca/content/dam/dalhousie/pdf/library/CoreSkills/6_Criteria_for_Websites.pdf)

These criteria are:

1. Does the agency, person, or institution that created the website have the **authority** to present information? What are their knowledge and qualifications to address the issue?
2. What is the **purpose** of the website? Does it provide the answers it proposes to address?
3. What is the **coverage** of the website? Are the topics explored in depth and is it comprehensive?
4. How **current** is the information presented? When was it first posted and when was it last revised? These dates should be easy to find.
5. How **objective** is the information provided? Is there bias in the way the content is presented and is the site trying to sell you something?
6. How **accurate** is the information on the website? Are there statistics to support the facts they present? Is the author part of a respectable institution and is the website written with correct grammar and spelling (a sure sign of an amateur website)?

Other tips include:

*   Look for websites from established institutions such as the American Cancer Society or The Centers for Disease Control and Prevention
*   Be careful with commercial sites that often try to sell a miracle cure
*   If the website does not tell you the name of the author or have a 'contact us' feature, be careful evaluating what they present

Adele continued her search on the internet, but now with a more critical eye. She found the most useful information from websites from large comprehensive cancer centers; there was information tailored for patients and families that she found easy to read and that presented a lot of factual information. She printed out the pages and put them into a color-coded binder. She pressed Norman to read the articles, but he was not interested.

"I want to hear things from the horse's mouth, Adele", he told her one morning over breakfast. "One of the guys who's working on the shopping mall we're building, you know where that is, anyway he said that his father had the same cancer as Jonathan and I'm meeting him for coffee later".

"Oh, that sounds good. We can talk about what he told you at dinner. Should I invite the kids?"

Norman was not sure that Jonathan should hear what the older man would tell him but as usual, he left the decision with his wife. Adele called Jonathan who said he was busy that evening but Sylvie and Matt were pleased that they didn't have to cook dinner.

Norman looked unhappy when he arrived from work later that day. Adele had made a lovely dinner for them, but Norman barely touched his food as he reported what the elderly father of is employee told him.

"Mr Harrison, that's the guy's name, must be close to 80, but I didn't ask him how old he is. He told me that he was diagnosed about 10 years ago and he said that he wished he had refused the surgery and rather let the cancer take its course! He showed me his bag and honestly, I almost threw up right there in the coffee shop".

Norman was visibly upset.

"Maybe we need a second opinion for Jonathan. He just agreed to the first thing offered by the surgeon and well, surgeons like to cut, don't they?"

"Hang on a minute, Dad!" Sylvie didn't want to hear anymore about this old man and his experience. "That was 10 years ago! Things have changed in medicine…."

"Your daughter is right!" Adele wanted to shut down the conversation before she started to doubt what Jonathan had decided.

"I've been reading stuff on the web and this surgeon has a really good reputation. And the hospital is one of the best in the country! Jonathan has faith in this guy, and we have to support him!"

"But ... this guy, the old guy, went through the same thing!"

"No Dad, he may not have! Do you even know that Jonathan's cancer is the same as his?"

Dr Katz advises:

While it may appear helpful to ask someone else with cancer about their experience, it is important to note that what someone else went through, may not apply to your family member. People often don't recall the details of their disease; the grade and stage of the cancer may be very different, and the outcomes of the treatment may be different too. With colorectal cancer, the site of the cancer may be anywhere in the intestines, all the way to the anal canal. The treatments for these cancers will differ and treatments themselves have changed over time as new techniques and medications have been developed.

Personal stories and more recently, blogs by people who have gone through cancer treatment as well as testimonials on social media, represent one person's experience. This does not necessarily translate to another individual whose own life experience will impact on how they cope with treatment.

Young adults use social media to connect to others and to feel less alone while dealing with the cancer. This can be helpful as it creates community; talking to others who are facing the same challenges, even if they don't have the same kind of cancer, can make things more bearable. Support groups are a well-established way that individuals can meet others with the same kind of cancer. They may be facilitated by a professional such as a nurse or social worker, or they may be peer-led. One of the challenges for young adults with cancer is that participants in these support groups are usually much older and do not face the same issues that a young adult may. Support groups for young adults with cancer may not be available in all areas and this is where online support groups can be helpful, no matter where the person lives or receives care.

Norman shook his head; he didn't know the details of the older man's cancer, and the man himself seemed to be confused about the details. Perhaps speaking to the man was not as helpful as he thought it was going to be.

"Okay, okay. I'm going to try and forget what he told me", Norman gave in with grace. "What we now must do is support Jonathan without question and without voicing our opinions. Can we agree on that?"

"Sure, honey. Of course. That was what we were all trying to do ..." Adele jumped in first.

"Amen" was Matt's response; he usually let the others do the talking and just observed the family dynamics.

"About damn time!" muttered Sylvie under her breath.

Conclusion

Family members need to support the individual with cancer in any way they can, taking into account the needs and desires of their family member. Their own needs for support are often relegated to the backburner and they may find it difficult to ask for and access help and support. Parents and partners often try to be the 'information finders' for the person with cancer and this can lead to misinformation if they don't use reliable sources. There are many different organizations and associations that provide support for people with cancer and their families; these range from valid information to financial assistance and also emotional and practical support. A list of resources is provided at the end of this chapter.

Reflective Questions

After reading this story:

- How could Jonathan's mother have better supported him rather than presenting questionable information about unproven treatment?
- What resources have YOU found helpful when seeking out information about cancer?
- How can you balance the opinions of various family members with the plan that the person with cancer has chosen?
- What are the pros and cons of finding information on the internet?

Resources

Books

Katz, A. (2014). *This Should Not Be Happening: Young Adults with Cancer.*
Hygeia Media.
Katz, A. (2015). *Meeting the Need for Psychosocial Care in Young Adults with Cancer.* Oncology Nursing Society.

Websites

National Cancer Institute
https://www.cancer.gov/types/aya
Cancer.Net
https://www.cancer.net/navigating-cancer-care/
young-adults-and-teenagers/being-young-adult-or-teen-with-cancer
American Cancer Society
https://www.cancer.org/cancer/cancer-in-young-adults.html
Canadian Cancer Society
https://www.cancer.ca/en/search/?q=YOUNG+ADULT

Patient Support Organizations

Livestrong
https://www.livestrong.org/we-can-help/young-adults
https://www.livestrong.org/we-can-help/just-diagnosed/
young-adults-with-cancer
Stupid Cancer
https://stupidcancer.org/
Cancer Fight Club
https://cancerfightclub.com/
Teen Cancer America
https://teencanceramerica.org/
First Descents
https://firstdescents.org/
Cactus Cancer Society
https://cactuscancer.org/
Testicular Cancer Society
https://testicularcancersociety.org/

Young Survivor Coalition
https://www.youngsurvival.org/
Critical Mass
https://www.criticalmass.org/
FuckCancer
https://www.letsfcancer.com/
Whole Lotta Life Foundation
https://wholelottalife.org/
Imerman Angels
https://imermanangels.org/
The Samfund
http://www.thesamfund.org/
Ulman Foundation
https://ulmanfoundation.org/
Leukemia & Lymphoma Society of Canada
https://www.llscanada.org/resources-for-parents-caregivers

Practical Support

Lotsa Helping Hands
https://lotsahelpinghands.com/
CaringBridge
https://www.caringbridge.com
Family Patient Online Patient Update Reports
www.familypatient.com
MyLifeLine
https://www.mylifeline.org

INDEX

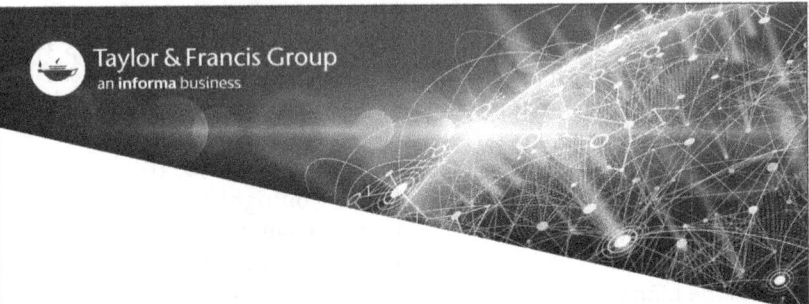
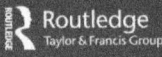
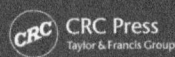